REALISTIC WEIGHT CONTROL

Jan de Vries was born in Holland in 1937 and grew up in occupied territory during the difficult war years. Graduating in pharmacy, he turned to alternative medicine. His most influential teacher was Dr Alfred Vogel in Switzerland, and they have worked together closely for 35 years.

In 1970 he and his family moved to Scotland and settled in Troon where he set up a residential clinic. He also has clinics in Newcastle, Edinburgh and London. He lectures throughout the world and is a regular broadcaster on BBC radio. His books have sold over a quarter of a million copies to date.

Books available from the same author

By Appointment Only series

Arthritis, Rheumatism and Psoriasis (second edition)
Asthma and Bronchitis
Cancer and Leukaemia (second edition)
Heart and Blood Circulatory Problems
Migraine and Epilepsy (fourth impression)
The Miracle of Life
Multiple Sclerosis (second edition)
Neck and Back Problems (second edition)
Skin Diseases
Stomach and Bowel Disorders
Stress and Nervous Disorders (second edition, second impression)
Traditional Home and Herbal Remedies (second edition)
Viruses, Allergies and the Immune System (fourth impression)
Who's Next? (second edition)

Nature's Gift series

Body Energy
Food
Water - Healer or Poison?

Well Woman series

Menopause
Menstrual and Pre-menstrual Tension

The Jan de Vries Healthcare series

Questions and Answers on Family Health
Life Without Arthritis - the Maori Way

REALISTIC WEIGHT CONTROL

THE HEALTHY GUIDE TO WEIGHT LOSS

JAN DE VRIES

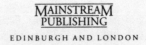

MAINSTREAM
PUBLISHING

EDINBURGH AND LONDON

This edition 1994

First published in Great Britain in 1989 by
MAINSTREAM PUBLISHING COMPANY (EDINBURGH) LTD
7 Albany Street
Edinburgh EH1 3UG

ISBN 1 85158 650 4

A catalogue record for this book is available from the British Library

Typeset in 11/13 pt Palatino by Polyprint, Edinburgh
Printed in Great Britain by Biddles Ltd, Guildford and King's Lynn

This book is dedicated to
my wife, Joyce,
without whose help
it would never have been written.

"Beauty and vitality are the gifts of Nature for those who live according to her law."
Leonardo da Vinci

Contents

Preface

EVER SINCE I was a child I have always been amazed by the terrific problems experienced by those who are overweight. Thirty years ago, when working in a pharmacy in Holland, I became aware of the tremendous sales of slimming products, particularly when a special window display was mounted featuring slimming products in order to boost sales during a quiet period. There never failed to be an increase in turnover if special attention was given to this colossal problem.

Later on in life, as a practitioner, I saw how a lot of money was spent in our residential clinics with a view to controlling excess weight. Faced with this huge demand for courses of dieting, fasting, and sometimes hammering one's body to get this extra weight off, I often wondered why this should be so; during the war I had seen people dying of hunger and I myself, at the age of ten, weighed only two and a half stones. The answer soon became clear and it is something we all have to realise: only by overeating can one expect this problem of excess weight. In today's society, particularly in view of all the convenience foods people are using, the naturopathic view — a realistic approach to dieting — has become of great importance.

It goes beyond description how I battle daily with this problem of obesity with my patients, and how much better they feel when they lose their excess weight. The mind is sharper, the body feels better; yet despite this they can easily fall into the trap of overeating again, and then torture themselves with methods which perhaps might be unhealthy, in an effort to try and lose the excess weight yet again. Despite all the efforts of slimming clinics, slimming diets, and even some more irresponsible methods, patients persistently damage their own health. When there is no balance between protein, carbohydrates and fats, people become victims of certain illnesses and diseases.

In this book we will go through a number of different and responsible methods of slimming. Having dealt with this problem for almost thirty years, I have seen the side-effects caused by irresponsible methods. Therefore, when people turn to our slimming department for help, we try, in a logical way, to bring their weight under control. It is a wonderful thing when a patient who was previously four or five stones overweight comes to you and, having successfully lost this weight, tells you that life has a new meaning for her. She feels so much happier, so much more beautiful and, having lost her corpulence, feels a part of society again. So many fall by the wayside, and that is where the greatest problems arise. It is a matter of continuing the treatment, which, as we have worked it out, is really not complicated. The results will not be visible overnight, but the ultimate reward, mentally and physically, is of the greatest importance.

The simple methods described in this book will be of the greatest assistance in what, for so many people, is a great battle. Just think of the words of Robert the Bruce, when, alone and dejected, he was hiding from his enemies in a cave and observed the perseverance of a spider in its attempts to build a web. When it finally reached its goal, he said: "If at first you don't succeed, try, try, try again!"

1

Do You Really Want to Lose Weight?

THERE ARE FEW conditions afflicting the human body
that cause more distress than fat, all the more so because
the sufferer knows that in most cases it is of his or her
own making. People with a physical handicap or illness
causing distortion of the body or features can hold their
heads up in the knowledge that fate has dealt them
an unfortunate blow, but the obese person suffers the
humiliation of knowing that his or her own weakness is
apparent for all to see.

Many people go through life "playing" at diets. One
week it's the 1,000-calorie diet; the week after that sees
the start of the vegetarian diet . . . followed by the low-
calorie diet and then the very low-calorie diet. Eventually
comes the water fast. Unfortunately, at the end of all this
dieting, the dieter finds that nothing has worked. The life
of a "playing at diets" dieter proceeds as follows:

Monday morning. Mrs X stands up. Today is the day for
a new diet. Strengthened with a cup of black coffee and
enthusiasm, she starts her daily work. By eleven o'clock,

13

visions of food loom large on the horizon. By twelve o'clock, hallucinations have set in, her blood sugar being so low that her body no longer can function.

After a lunch of lettuce, cottage cheese and perhaps a tomato, Mrs X continues with her daily work, but something is not quite right. Perhaps a cup of tea with a little digestive biscuit might help. Yes, much better. But maybe another digestive biscuit, because, after all, not much has been eaten today.

After several more digestive biscuits, Mrs X comes to the conclusion that the diet has failed again. Come teatime, everything in sight is eaten. After tea, settling down to a nice cosy evening by the television with the usual drinks, nuts, crisps and sweets, Mrs X looks back over her day. She finds she hasn't done badly. After all, she managed up until about two o'clock. Oh well, it's too late now to start this week. Next Monday we'll do better!

This sounds amusing, but is it? Do you recognise yourself? Many people who deviate from their diet, even slightly, become discouraged and stop altogether. These are the "playing at dieting" dieters. Very often, however, there is an underlying reason for this.

Some people just *think* they want to be slim, but deep down they feel that being slim will give them responsibilities which they do not have to bear now. Perhaps they find it difficult to accompany their partner on social occasions. Perhaps being looked at with admiration is too much for them. Even the thought of having a different physical appearance is frightening for some people. Therefore, it's easier to just pretend to diet, to say you're dieting, even believe you're dieting. You may even manage to persuade yourself that you *want* to diet, that you *want* to be slim, but, alas, experience has taught you that you were meant to be fat and that your metabolism is different from everybody else's — in spite of what the doctor says, yours goes at a much slower rate than the norm.

So it follows that your lot in life is to be fat, not to be attractive, not to be so lucky as some people and have an attractive figure . . . and go places . . . and do things. The world is geared towards self-confident, slim people — not towards fatties like you!

This is the way that many people with a weight problem think. They forget their beautiful hair, their lovely eyes, their fine skin or their high intelligence. All they can see is this great fat mound of flesh. Whether it be half a stone or several stones, it is still a problem.

Some dieters think that their friend's half a stone of excess weight is nothing. They'll tell her, "I wouldn't worry if I were you. If I were like that, I'd be happy." Unfortunately, it doesn't work like this. Half a stone is just as distressing as several stones. It is still excess weight, it is unattractive, it is confidence undermining and it should not be there.

Laying aside for the moment the physical discomforts which accompany being overweight, just think of the mental ones: this feeling of having to apologise for one's existence, this feeling of inferiority, of self-consciousness. These attitudes really do undermine everything that an overweight person does.

Without losing an ounce, you can do a lot to help yourself. Stand up straight. There, you've already lost half a stone. Think about what you're wearing. Dress to flatter your figure — big can be beautiful. Look the whole world in the face. Why should you be self-conscious? You're you. Why should you feel inferior? You're not. Don't be arrogant or defensive. There is no reason for arrogance, nor is there any reason for defensiveness. Be friendly and be obliging and you'll find that however you react to the world will be reflected in its attitude towards you.

Now, let's get back to this question: do you really want to lose weight?

Medical science has proved that people who constantly lose and gain weight are not doing their body any good. It is healthier to maintain a constant weight, even if it is too much. Remember, whatever weight you are, you're you. Your character remains the same; your faults and failures remain the same, and so do your strengths. The only difference is that you look and feel healthier. Don't think that your personality will change or that all your troubles will disappear because you've lost weight. Admittedly, that feeling of depression will almost certainly go, leaving you feeling much happier, but basically you will still be the same person.

Having weighed up the pros and cons of losing or not losing weight, and having made your decision, abide by it. Should you have decided not to lose weight, then don't dwell upon it — forget your weight. Instead, concentrate on your strong points. Concentrate on being attractive. Think "big is beautiful". It can be, you know. Remember, though, it is also a health hazard: if you are more than 20 per cent overweight, then your health may be at risk.

Obesity tends to occur more frequently in women than in men, and more so in middle-aged women than in young women. It can cause, among other things, diabetes, nephritis, pneumonia, miocardial failure, degenerative arthritis of the back of the knees, foot trouble, varicose veins and leg ulcers — to say nothing of the possible complications which might arise during surgery.

The risk of dying between the ages of forty-five and fifty is 8 per cent higher than average for people who are ten pounds overweight. This rises to 18 per cent for those who are twenty pounds and 28 per cent for those who are thirty pounds overweight. Finally, if you are fifty pounds overweight, the chance of your dying before you reach the age of fifty is an alarming 56 per cent higher than if you were of normal weight. Perhaps if your own vital statistics have not succeeded in persuading you to lose weight, then these will.

Sometimes obesity is familial, that is, every member of a family will be overweight — some more, some less, but overweight nevertheless. The reason for this is not as might be expected, slow metabolism, but usually bad eating habits. Mother cooks large meals which are duly consumed and appreciated by her family. Then the children get married. Daughters, anxious to impress new husbands, cook huge meals which are also duly appreciated . . . and so it goes on . . . generation after generation of portly family members.

When the younger generation complain about being overweight, then they are consoled by the older ones who say, "Oh well, look at the stock you come from. You can't expect to be thin. We were born fat. We were always fat. We are just built this way." And so, the young person consoles herself with yet another packet of crisps, and philosophically sits back to ensure an unhappy and fat adulthood.

Whatever the reason for obesity, the cause is always the same: too much food. Some people can consume a great amount of food and not gain weight. Others consume very little and still seem to put on weight. However, without eating too much, for you personally, you will not gain weight.

You might say, "Look at my neighbour. She eats the whole day long and she's not in the least bit fat." Indeed, look at your neighbour. She is perhaps a lot thinner than you are — but look, too, at her lifestyle. Is she very active? Does she run around the whole day while you sit? Does she go to gymnastics and aerobics classes or go swimming while you sit around watching the television or reading a book?

Recently, while dining out, I have been secretly observing other diners. Some were fat, some were thin, some were of average weight. However, I noticed a marked difference in their eating habits. The thinner people tended to do a lot of talking and not quite so much eating. They put their fork down between each mouthful, savouring and enjoying what they were eating. Their larger companions, on the other hand, shovelled in the food as quickly as they could and were finished long before their thin companions.

17

I also noticed a difference in their choices from the menu. The more corpulent people enjoyed thick soups, rich sauces and creamy desserts, while their thinner companions tended to choose consommé to start with, followed by a salad and then fresh fruit or fresh fruit salad. Both parties were consuming the same number of courses. Both parties had full plates. However, the total number of calories on one plate was very different to that on the other.

Many slim people will tell you that they have great appetites — that they are constantly eating. Yet I have noticed with such people that they tend to prefer the sort of food that will not give them an obese figure. Their preference tends towards vegetables, fruit, brown bread, baked potatoes, very little fat, and lean meat.

These people are lucky. Their natural choice of food is non-addictive and non-fattening. They will not overeat because, although they enjoy what they are eating, it is not the sort of food that one does over-indulge in. Also, it is the sort of food that one eats sitting at a table during mealtimes. These types also tend not to nibble between meals. A cup of coffee is sufficient, or a cup of tea, and nothing else is necessary.

Often these habits have been laid down during childhood. If a child is discouraged from eating rubbish, then he or she will grow up to be an adult who prefers good food.

I am frequently consulted by a lady accompanied by a child, where the lady is very overweight but the child is of normal weight. Nevertheless the child will arrive in the consulting-room with a packet of crisps or sweets. If I remark upon this, then the lady will say, "Oh, he has nothing to worry about. Look how thin he is." She is then very surprised when I reply, "Yes, he's thin now, but actually by encouraging your child to eat this sort of food, you are storing up for him a fat future and the same sort of misery as you are now going through yourself." The usual reaction to this is sheer disbelief. The lady very often becomes indignant at the very thought that she might be teaching her child bad habits.

Children who are given food as a reward frequently grow up to be tubby teenagers and fat adults. Habits acquired in childhood can be life-long, but they need not be so. Such habits have been made and therefore they can be unmade, or broken.

Most young mothers are surprised at the manner in which their young babies consume food. A very young child or baby will not overeat: it knows when it has had enough and no amount of coaxing by adults will persuade it to allow one more drop of milk in its mouth than is necessary. This can cause alarm in adults because some children can survive on very little and yet remain completely healthy.

As time progresses, the child learns to enjoy treats. These are given by the parents, fond aunties and even fonder grandparents. The types of food given as treats are usually addictive. Crisps and sweets can be eaten in any amount and very often a child comes to prefer these non-nutritious foods to the food presented at the table — food that is nourishing and essential for a young, growing body.

So often do I get in my consulting-room young women or men who are very unhealthy. They are fat and they are flabby. When questioned about their eating habits, they admit that they do not like milk, they do not like potatoes and they do not like brown bread. Instead, they consume large amounts of fish and chips, lemonade and white bread and jam, and are quite happy. Those are what they have been taught from early childhood to enjoy as treats and those are what they now choose to eat rather than proper food.

If they wish to lose weight, such people will have to review their eating habits and they will have to drastically change them. In order to become slim, trim and healthy a whole new lifestyle must be adopted.

As I have said, just as bad habits have been learned, they can also be unlearned. It is not easy. It takes a certain amount of will-power and a certain amount of determination. It also takes time. If a person realises this and is willing to try, then it is possible. Lifestyles can be reviewed and renewed as often as is necessary.

Having read what I have said about being overweight and having decided that you really want to lose weight, then read on. Make up your mind that this time you will succeed. No more yo-yoing up and down. You're going to lose weight and you're going to lose it permanently. You're not going to gain weight again because you're going to learn how to control it. You're going to learn how to eat for health and discover that life can be just as happy and just as fulfilling without all the stodge, the sweet things, the fat, and the fizzy drinks. You're going to learn how to live a new life and you're going to find that it is a much more abundant one.

2

Reasons for Being Overweight

AS HAS BEEN said, the only reason why anybody is overweight is that they consume more food than their particular body can use. If you can imagine your body as a fire that is burning fuel in order to function, then you can see what happens and how the way in which you burn this fuel can affect its efficiency. The fuel used by the body is calories. Calories measure heat, one calorie being the amount of heat needed to raise one cubic centimetre of water by one degree centigrade.

Now, this is not a very useful way of measuring, so we tend to talk about calories when we really mean kilocalories, which refer to the amount of heat required to raise the temperature of one litre of water by one degree centigrade. In more recent times, units of heat have also been expressed in kilojoules for scientific purposes, but in this book I will talk about calories, though I really mean kilocalories.

Calories are burned up when the body performs such basic functions as breathing, digesting and maintaining a heart beat and body temperature; in other words, merely by keeping us alive. The rate at which you burn calories while doing absolutely nothing except existing is called your Basic Metabolic Rate, or BMR. Maintaining your basic functions requires two-thirds of your daily calorie intake. The average woman has a BMR of just under 60 calories per hour, whereas that of the average man is just under 70 calories per hour.

Moving about increases our metabolism. Therefore it will be clear that the more active we are, the more calories we are going to burn and the higher our metabolism will be.

The only organ in our body which does not use calories, unfortunately, is our brain. However mentally active we are, the more we sit about thinking, the fewer calories we will burn by doing physical things. As the world becomes increasingly computerised, and as more and more people tend to have sedentary jobs, we are finding that we require less food.

For example, think of the level of physical activity involved in just one aspect of modern housekeeping — washing the clothes. Everything is mechanical: press a button and your washing is done; press another button and it's dry. The only really physical activity required on washing day is the ironing. Now consider the same task as it was performed about 100 years ago. Think of the boilerhouse: the washing had to be boiled and it had to be stamped. There was a washboard which had to be used. Then it had to be put through the wringer — the mangle. All this required a great amount of effort, and many calories were used up in the process.

I remember my mother telling me about washing day when she was young. My grandmother used to do her washing on a Monday. This really began on Sunday evening, when the whole family would sit around the fire preparing vegetables for the next day's broth. While they were doing that, my grandmother would mix the ingredients for a steamed pudding. Both were put on the hob before retiring to bed in the evening and simmered gently the whole night through and during the following morning, leaving her the opportunity to get on with her washing.

Come lunchtime, everything would be ready: a nice thick broth full of lentils or barley and vegetables, with a good shank of meat in it, followed by a heavy steamed pudding filled with lard. The family was not fat, but then all of them had manual jobs. All of them required a great number of calories in order to keep their bodies healthy.

Today, there are still people who eat like that; they have carried on the family tradition and then wonder why they are overweight. Yet it should be remembered that we live in a different day and age. We are not nearly so active. If we want to be active, we have to go and look for activity. We have to join swimming clubs or aerobics classes. This is the sort of activity that the modern person pursues.

However, such activities are self-limiting, because most of them take place after working hours. These are our leisure hours and we do not always want to spend our leisure hours doing something physical. Sometimes we feel we are too tired and sometimes there are other things to do — things that do not require many calories. In this case we have to consume less food in order to accommodate our lifestyle.

Unfortunately, most people acquire their dietary patterns in their teenage years. These years are the most active years of our lives. When we are at school there are games; then there is dancing . . . all sorts of things to burn up calories. Later, there is a busy social life to get through. Later still, young women get married and have children. These children are very active and a great amount of energy is required in order to look after them. Later still, these children grow up and are able to do things for themselves, and their mother does not have nearly such a busy job. But what is she eating? Exactly the same as she ate when she was a teenager.

Thus you can see why it is that women come to complain about their middle-age spread. In fact, there is no such thing as a middle-age spread. What has really happened is that the mother has not, in her middle years, adjusted her diet to suit her new lifestyle.

Now I will return to the Basic Metabolic Rate or BMR. When talking about this I used the word "average" — 60 calories for women, 70 calories for men. Unfortunately, there is no such thing as the average woman or the average man, so these figures are not the laws of the Medes and the Persians. They have to be adjusted to suit the individual.

It is, in fact, possible to find out what an individual's metabolic rate is. This can be done professionally using a piece of apparatus which is completely sealed and contains air. The person whose metabolic rate we want to find breathes in and out of this container. The apparatus also contains a chemical which absorbs carbon dioxide, the gas we expel when we breathe out. Gradually, the volume of air in the container decreases because of the oxygen used in breathing. By measuring this deficit, it is possible to calculate the number of calories used in just existing. This must be done, as has been said, by an expert. There is, however, a much more easily available do-it-yourself method, which will tell you how your BMR relates to that of the "average" person, or the norm.

The norm is taken to be a man weighing 70 kilograms wearing indoor clothing, and measuring 1.7 metres, who uses an average of 1,700 calories in twenty-four hours, provided that he has an empty stomach and is sitting in a room heated to a temperature of 20° centigrade. This is the average BMR for a man; that for a woman is about 10 per cent less.

First of all, you must find out your blood pressure. Ask your doctor to tell you what it is. Having received this information, sit down and relax. When you are quite sure that you are as relaxed as possible, count your pulse rate and make a note of it. In order to work out your deviation from the norm, you then apply this information to the following formula:

If f is the pulse rate, and a is the difference between the systolic and diastolic blood pressure readings, then

$$\tfrac{2}{3}\,(f + a) - 72$$

will give you the deviation from the norm.

Let us put this into figures. For example, if $f = 80$ and $a = 50$, then we get:

$$\tfrac{2}{3}\,(80 + 50) - 72 = 87 - 72.$$
$$= 15.$$

This means that you deviate 14 per cent from the norm. Deviations of up to 20 per cent are quite normal.

(Remember, when you take the necessary readings the room temperature must be 20° centigrade and you must also have an empty stomach.)

In order to lose weight, then, one must consume fewer calories than are necessary to keep this BMR going. Many people will tell me that they cannot lose weight when on a 1,000-calorie diet. This I find very difficult to believe. When I question such people further about their diet they will tell me, "Oh yes, I stick to 1,000 calories per day", and they will proceed to describe what they eat. Then when I ask them how much of it they are eating, they look blank. Obviously, in order to count 1,000 calories, one must measure and weigh the food.

Often, in my consulting-room, the dialogue goes as follows:

Me: "Tell me, now, what do you eat in a day?"
Dieter: "Oh, I start the morning with a bowl of cereal with some milk in it and some fruit juice. Then for my lunch I have a piece of cheese and a piece of bread with an apple, and then in the evening . . . oh, just meat and a potato and veg. And that's it."
Me: "Right. Let's get back to the morning. How much cereal do you take?"
Dieter: "Oh, not much. Just a wee bowl."
Me: "Mm. How much milk goes into it?"

Dieter: "Not much. Just enough."

Me: "Right. What about lunchtime then? How much bread do you take?"

Dieter: "Just a slice."

Me: "How much did the bread weigh? How many calories were in it?"

Dieter: "Sixty."

Me: "How do you know?"

Dieter: "Oh, well, it was just a wee slice."

Me: "Mm. Did you have butter on it?"

Dieter: "Yes."

Me: "Yes, right. What did you have for elevenses?"

Dieter: "Oh yes, a cup of coffee."

Me: "Milk and sugar?"

Dieter: "Yes, yes."

Me: "Did you count the calories?"

Dieter: "Oh, it was just a wee drop."

Me: "Right. The next thing is teatime."

Dieter: "Yes?"

Me: "What did you have? How much meat did you have?"

Dieter: "Oh, not much."

Me: "How many potatoes?"

Dieter: "Oh, just one or two."

Me: "What did you have after your main meal?"

Dieter: "Yoghurt."

Me: "How much?"

Dieter: "Just a tub."

Me: "Flavoured?"

Dieter: "Yes."

Me: "How many calories?"

Dieter: "Oh, just a tub of yoghurt."

Me: "Did you have anything during the evening?"

Dieter: "Not much, just a drink, a biscuit. You know, just the usual — not much."

Me: "And you had 1,000 calories?"

Dieter: "Yes, yes, I had 1,000 calories."

Me: "How do you know?"

Dieter: "Oh well, I didn't eat much."

You will realise, of course, that what this dieter consumed could be any number of calories. What is a lot for one is very little for another, as amounts are relative. The only way to find out exactly how many calories you are consuming is to weigh everything you eat. For this reason I do not recommend a 1,000-calorie diet to my patients. My diet sheets consist of foods and the amounts of them to be consumed, measured in ounces or grams.

Sloppiness will lead to unsuccessful weight loss. People will think that they are dieting, but unfortunately they are again just "playing" at dieting. In order to diet properly, you must be very aware of exactly what you are consuming.

To go back to what was said at the beginning of this chapter, the one and only reason for your being overweight is that you are consuming more calories than your body needs. Having said that, there are many reasons for this. These can be divided into two categories: *physical* factors and *psychological* factors.

These are now the reasons why it is so difficult to lose weight. If it were just a question of arithmetic, then anybody who was careful would lose weight; but, alas, will-power comes into play here as well.

Let us look first at the *physical* factors. These are perhaps more easy to adjust. They also can be subdivided as follows:

(a) bad eating habits, individual or familial;
(b) ignorance;
(c) being too busy.

If one of these is truly the reason for your fat, then the solution is easy — education! All that is necessary is to be given a good diet and for you to adhere to it. If you are willing to be taught, if the person teaching you is a responsible person and if the diet is good, then there will be no problem. Be advised, do what you are told, learn from it and you will find that your weight will disappear quite easily.

The next category of people is more difficult. Their problem is *psychological* in origin. It is not so easy for them to follow a diet and experience success. There are many psychological reasons for being overweight:

    (a) insecurity;
    (b) boredom;
    (c) loneliness;
    (d) worry;
    (e) night-eating;
    (f) appetite rather than hunger;
    (g) influence of advertising.

In order to overcome these difficulties, you must first be aware of them. Then, you must identify the situations when you are most tempted. Having done that and having analysed the difficult times, then the next step is to work out a "plan of campaign". You must realise that the problem does exist and do something positive about it.

Unfortunately, most people with a psychological factor controlling their eating consider themselves to be unique. They believe that they are the only ones with a problem and think that if they were in different circumstances and had a different set of problems, then it would be much easier.

How often have I come across a lady in my consulting-room lamenting the fact that since she came to be alone in the world her problem has increased. And how often have I heard her sigh, "I wish I had somebody to share my life with. Then things would be much easier."

Equally often, another type of lady comes to my consulting-room. This time she is a mother of young children and has a husband who does shift-work. This lady has often given up a promising career in order to become a housewife. At first it's very exciting — there's a certain freedom — but soon she finds that there is something lacking in her life. She misses her colleagues; she misses the responsibility that she used to have and she finds that she feels trapped by four walls and a crowd of screaming children. This sends her to the food cupboard; she eats irresponsibly and then wonders why her weight level has changed. Her lament is, "Oh, if only I were on my own, then I would manage my eating much more easily."

The conclusion that I come to, listening to both extremes, is that there is no easy solution. One lady's problem is just as difficult to deal with as the other, although they are caused by opposing factors. One imagines that if she had a companion, she would manage her eating better. The other believes that if she had less company it would be much easier. There is no easy way; each person has to find what for them is the most successful manner in which to manage their life.

Just as I have grouped boredom and loneliness together, so, too, there is a connection between insecurity and worry. Both conditions also tend to send the sufferers to the food cupboard. The solution is the same: identify when the difficult times are likely to occur, face up to the fact, and plan to do something other than eating food at these difficult times.

This of course is very easily said, but not so easy to put into practice. People suffering from boredom, loneliness, insecurity or worry tend to succumb very easily to such bad habits as night-eating or bingeing. In order to break these habits then, you must be very strongly motivated. Remember, these habits were acquired by you, and the only one who can break them is yourself.

Some problems are easily solved. For example, if you find yourself being influenced by the advertisements on television, then turn over to a non-commercial channel. If you see people eating on television, and have a great desire to follow them, then don't watch such things.

Are you a night-eater? Don't worry about it: you can easily cope with this problem by spreading your daily diet over a 24-hour period. If you take into account the fact that you are going to wake in the night and look for something to eat, then see to it that something is there. See to it that you have kept something back that you could have eaten during the day, and then you will not spoil your diet and will still lose weight.

Many people do very well on a diet for a certain length of time and then suddenly something goes wrong. All they can think about is food, and this preoccupation will eventually lead them to eating it. Then one item is eaten after the other until they realise that they are on a full-blown binge. This can be extremely dangerous. Some people having had a binge, decide that the diet will not work, that all is lost, that they will never lose weight, so what's the use? As a result, the diet is given up. For others the solution is more sinister. They decide that having eaten all that food, it must be got rid of and got rid of quickly, so they go into the toilet and force themselves to vomit. Now this particular practice is very habit-forming and can eventually lead to the condition of anorexia nervosa or bulimia nervosa, which can lead to hospitalisation and even death. So you must be very, very careful.

If you have read this far, then you have obviously decided that you really do want to lose weight. The problems I have touched upon will be further and more closely examined in later chapters; so read carefully, and you will find a solution for your particular problem.

3

Temptation

OF ALL THE afflictions impeding the progress of a dieter, the most difficult to deal with is temptation. It creeps up unawares, then suddenly something sparks off the thought and the mind becomes obsessed with finding something to eat.

Let us look at what Mrs X is doing:

It's Monday again. Mrs X has started a new diet and, as the day goes on, is keeping to it beautifully. At about three o'clock she sits down with a cup of tea — nothing to eat, mind!

Switching on the television, she is confronted immediately by a beautiful girl biting into a lovely, gooey Mars bar. Feeling very superior she continues to sip her tea, but, alas, the seed has been sown.

She finishes watching the commercials, but her mind is no longer on them. Somewhere, somehow, the only things she can think of are Mars bars.

Switching off the television she picks up a book. After reading a page or two, she realises that she has no idea what she has been reading. At the back of her mind her subconscious is busy, and it keeps on saying "Mars bars!".

She decides that something constructive must be done and so she starts to do some ironing, but all the while she has visions of Mars bars. If only she hadn't been so virtuous. If only she hadn't cleaned out all her cupboards so that there was nothing left to eat. Is there nothing left? What's in the fridge?

Leaving the ironing, she goes and looks in the fridge and finds nothing. Surely there's something somewhere! The bread bin and the store cupboard are just as she had left them. They contain only the bare necessities. Opening the freezer she finds ice-cream. Ah, the very thing. Not quite a Mars bar, but it will do in the meantime!

Temptation can hit you suddenly, and lead to many negative emotions. It can lead to bingeing, it can cause depression, it can cause guilt and it can cause loss of self-respect, to name but a few.

What can a poor dieter do now, in order to resist temptation? Look at Mrs X again. Think of her actions. She was doing fine until she switched on the television. She knew that commercials usually involve food. Had she thought in advance, she would first of all have switched the television to a non-commercial channel before settling down.

Finding herself unable to concentrate on her book, she switched to ironing instead. Ironing is never the most stimulating of occupations and so her thoughts were free to wander. What did they settle on? Mars bars!

Now, whenever Mrs X is in this frame of mind it would be a good idea for her to take herself up to her bedroom and have a good long look at herself in the mirror. She could look at her rolls of fat and tell herself that these have been laid down because of her liking for Mars bars. In other words, they are self-afflicted.

Dwelling too long on this truth tends to be counter-productive, so, having taken a good look at herself, Mrs X could then start thinking positively. How would she look without the rolls of fat, and how could she achieve this state? While she is looking in the mirror anyway, how would she look with her hair up, or curled, or put to one side? Before long, Mrs X would be deeply engrossed in thoughts of the future.

Anyone who experiences problems with dieting knows what temptation is. Nearly everybody has had the experience of being on the point of succumbing to temptation when the telephone has rung or the doorbell has gone. The distraction caused by dealing with this invariably makes one forget whatever one was about to give in to.

Temptation is not always with us. If we can find an occupation which is distracting enough, then we can forget temptation. It will leave us alone. However, you must plan in advance, knowing that temptation will surely come. Write a list of stimulating occupations, then, when you feel tempted, look at it. It's no good trying to think of something in the middle of temptation because then nothing appeals. When one is tempted, the only thing that one wants to do, the only thing that is in one's mind, is succumbing to that temptation. So, when the very seed of it starts to grow, run to your list of occupations, choose one and think about it deeply. Submerge yourself in it and you will find that this seed of temptation will have died before it could take root.

Some people find that cleaning their teeth is a great help in getting rid of temptation. The clean taste of toothpaste tends to take away that feeling of wanting to eat something that one shouldn't. Physical activity is another good distractor. Many people who have taken up jogging have found that, when they come back even after a short jog, food is the last thing on their mind.

These are just a few suggestions. What helps one person does not necessarily help another. It's a case of trial and error. Try everything; find the thing that helps you the best, and then stick to it. If you still feel really tempted, try waiting twenty minutes before you succumb. Tell yourself, "I won't eat it for twenty minutes". In the meantime, find something to distract yourself and when the twenty minutes have passed the likelihood of the temptation also having passed is great.

The place where one is most easily tempted, of course, is in the kitchen. So, keep out of it as much as possible. Try not to be a taster. A little food is very moreish.

These are just small points but, remember, each little thing that makes it easier is one step in the right direction. Each pound that you lose must be worked for, so don't despise it. Don't think at the end of a week, after having lost just one pound, that it's not worth it. Remember, one pound per week adds up to almost four stones per year.

When I was young we used to sing a hymn at school which went like this:

> Yield not to temptation, for yielding is sin,
> Each victory will help you some other to win.

Now, I'm quite sure that whoever wrote this was not thinking about food at the time, but it is relevant just the same.

It may help to think of your mind as working like a computer. If you feed a basic programme for playing chess into a computer and then set a novice chess player against that computer, the novice chess player will win. After a few games, the player will find that he can no longer beat the computer. If you then set a moderately good player against the computer, that player, too, will win initially. Gradually, however, the computer will build up knowledge and, again, the chess player will begin to lose. Eventually the point will be reached where the computer will beat any professional, because, gradually, through doing things and through making mistakes, the computer will have built up a fund of knowledge that can confound anybody.

Now, if you apply this to your dieting and to dealing with your temptations, then you will find, just as the hymn writer says, "Each victory will help you some other to win".

4

Compulsion

THERE IS A SUBTLE difference between temptation and compulsion. When one is tempted, at the back of one's mind lurks some particular food that one wants to eat. With compulsion it is different. Very often there is no particular desire for one particular food. There is merely this feeling that one must put something, anything, in one's mouth.

Compulsion resembles a nervous habit like nail-biting. There is no particular pleasure to be gained from nail-biting. Yet the nail-biter must bite his nails. There is no rhyme or reason to it, just an instinct.

Compulsion, we can say then, is an instinct, an instinct that makes us constantly want to put something in our mouths. Babies have this instinct too. If they don't suck at the bottle or at the breast, then there is a tendency to suck the thumb. Elbow-bending, you see, is almost born in us!

There is a rare disease which compels the sufferer to stuff anything and everything in his mouth. Day and night this compulsion to eat anything and everything is present. Now, someone suffering from this disease, and luckily there are few of them, is doomed. There is no known cure. It causes brain damage and ultimately leads to death.

On a much smaller scale, compulsive eaters also do themselves much harm. We all know the experience of overloading our stomachs and finding it difficult to concentrate on something. The body cannot cope with clearing up all the rubbish we have eaten while still managing to keep our brains clear.

Compulsion hits suddenly with the full extent of its force, unlike temptation, which grows from a tiny seed. You've had a good meal, you're satisfied, you're not in the least bit hungry, but suddenly, this desire for something hits you. You don't really know what it is, and you start to look. Being diet conscious, you start with perhaps a grated carrot or, not having any time to grate a carrot because the compulsion is so great, a raw carrot. But that doesn't hit the spot. A digestive biscuit, then — very nice too, but still not right. And so you continue, gradually progressing from something comparatively innocent to the really high-calorie foods, yet still not being satisfied. You're full, in fact you're over full and feel ill because you have eaten so much, but still this urge to eat prevails.

This, now, is a real binge. Some bingers will go through the house picking at this and that until this urge to eat too much is finally satisfied. Others grab everything within sight that is edible and eat it. They don't really know what they're eating or how much of it they're eating; they go on, and on, and on, eating until they fall more or less comatose. Such bingers have been known to do themselves great bodily harm. They have had to be hospitalised, where they have had to have their stomachs pumped. On one or two occasions the bout of compulsive eating has even proved to be fatal.

As is the case with temptation, there are many reasons why a person should take to compulsive eating. Very often it is premenstrual tension. Many people tell stories of having kept nicely to their diets for three weeks before, all of a sudden, this urge to eat compulsively just hits them for no reason whatsoever. The problem here has often proved to be hormonal and medical help can be provided.

Sometimes the combination of all sorts of minor niggles become too much for people and the result is compulsive eating. Things are not going well in their marriage or at work, or they may be experiencing money worries, boredom, fear or anxiety. Some or all of these pressures can add up and suddenly become too much, and a bout of compulsive eating is triggered.

This indiscriminate eating of everything in sight is not the only sort of compulsive eating which occurs. Another kind resembles temptation in many ways, in that it is aimed at a certain food. Let's have a look at Mrs X again.

Poor Mrs X has been doing very well and is pleased with herself. She invites a friend to tea. The friend, alas, comes armed with, instead of a bunch of flowers, a beautiful box of chocolates. Mrs X enjoys her friend's company and does very well at the tea-table.

The friend departs and Mrs X puts the box of chocolates out of sight, telling herself that "out of sight is out of mind". Unfortunately for Mrs X, this turns out not to be the case. The box of chocolates is ever present in her mind. She tries various ways to get rid of this image, but the box of chocolates keeps hovering into view. At last she decides to open the box and just take one. Perhaps that will help.

This, of course, proves fatal. Before she knows where she is, Mrs X has eaten half the box and is still going strong. She's not hungry; she wasn't hungry when she started. She soon feels decidedly uncomfortable, but the only thing that she can think of is to empty that box, and then the temptation will be gone forever.

At last the box is empty and Mrs X feels decidedly ill. However, the temptation has gone, the box of chocolates has gone, and it's Thursday. She only needs to wait until Monday to start a new diet!

How often have you found yourself doing this too — giving in to this compulsion to empty whatever has been opened, be it a box of chocolates or the biscuit tin? This experience is different from temptation because when one is tempted one fights it all the way, even though sometimes it may be a losing battle. With compulsion, however, there is no thought of fighting it. It is just a compulsion: it has to be done, the food has to be got rid of and then the urge will be satisfied.

Sometimes temptation can turn into compulsion. I was once consulted by a lady who was very overweight. Her great weakness was chocolates — continental chocolates. One day she told me a sorry tale. She had been doing well in her diet and was loath to break it, when she received a beautiful box of expensive chocolates. She opened it, took one, and then decided that she was not going to be tempted any longer. Before she could think about it, she threw the box of chocolates in the dustbin outside. Feeling very satisfied with herself, she retired to bed.

At about two o'clock in the morning she woke up. She was feeling restless and suddenly remembered the box of chocolates. The desire for chocolate quickly overcame her. Mindlessly she went out to the dustbin on a dark blustery night, took out the remains of the box and scraped up the loose chocolates from the edges of the dustbin. There, still outside and beside all the rubbish, she consumed the rest!

It took a lot of courage on this lady's part to tell me this story. I'm glad to say that after much counselling and many ups and downs, the lady did manage to lose her excess weight. She managed to break this dreadful habit of compulsion and has now been slim for several years.

Her story reminds me of yet another lady who came to see me. This lady I saw twice, and I have often wondered what eventually happened to her. She, too, was extremely obese. I gave her the diet sheet and she departed enthusiastically. At her next consultation we found that she had actually gained two pounds, adding to what was already a considerable weight. When questioned, she broke down and told me that after having had a row with her boss one night, she had gone home and consumed five litres of Coca-Cola with four family-sized packets of potato crisps. She told me this as if it were the most ordinary thing in the world and I had difficulty in keeping a straight face because I didn't want to make her feel that she was an oddity. I managed to console her and she went away full of hope that she would do better the next time, but I never saw her again.

Now, this lady was really in need of psychiatric counselling. There appeared to be a deep psychological problem in her case that should really be dealt with by experts. Most dietary problems, although they are psychological, can be treated without the help of a psychiatrist, but this lady, I feel, was really on the verge of trouble.

Some people, through carelessness, compulsion, habit, or whatever, can reach an enormous size. One young man who came to see me was so heavy that I could not weigh him. My scales go up to twenty-six stones, but he still could not be weighed.

I advised this young man to stick to his diet and to measure himself and to be led by his inner self, that is, be very aware of how he was feeling. Within a short time I was able to register his weight. He told me that his problem was compulsive eating, but since receiving treatment and following the diet he had begun to feel much better. Seeing the inches coming off each time he measured himself, he had been undaunted by the fact that he could not be weighed. He was a happy man the day that the scales registered twenty-six stones and, since then, has gone on to lose several more stones and is still on the way down.

This young man was motivated and motivation is the true cure for compulsion. If you can just look inwardly, can just see and feel how much better you are mentally, spiritually and bodily, when you are adhering to a healthy diet, then this will be good motivation. But it is not the only motivation. If you are bored, then you will look for something to do, and what is easier than eating? So, if you try to keep busy, try to have something other than food at the forefront of your mind, then seeing the great improvement in yourself will help you keep going.

Remember, nothing breeds success like success.

5

Habits

LIKE MOST OTHER living beings, man is a creature of habit. We are always happiest when we are doing what we usually do. If we usually get up at seven o'clock in the morning and if we oversleep and rise at nine o'clock, we get a headache. Should eleven o'clock be our customary bedtime and we miss that, going to bed at twelve o'clock will see us shattered the next day. If we miss our coffee break in the morning, then there is a feeling that something is wrong.

Throughout the year we look forward to our holidays. When we are on holiday routine goes out of the window, but, secretly, we are looking forward to getting back and into our old routine. Habit is something very human.

Habits can be life-long, or they can be acquired along life's journey. We toilet train our children by cashing in on this habit-forming trait of human nature. Without understanding it, small children quickly form the habit of performing on a toilet at a given signal, or at a given time. Their bowels quickly learn to move every twenty-four hours because they have been trained to do so.

Think again of a young baby. This creature will drive other human beings to distraction, simply because it has no habits. They have not yet been formed. If a baby is wet or hungry, it will have no qualms whatsoever about arousing others in the middle of the night to see to it that it is made comfortable. Gradually, the parents instil some sort of routine into this little person's life, so that when it is convenient for them, then baby will be fed and changed.

Thinking along this line, it is easily understood that habits are life-long. Habits formed at a very early age will continue right through life. They are very necessary; if nobody had any habits then the world would be in chaos. If everybody started work when they felt like it, then no work would be done because nobody would be able to co-ordinate with anybody else. Everybody would be a complete and utter individual, living for himself alone.

We often speak about good habits and bad habits. When we think carefully about it, we find that good habits promote an orderly existence for ourselves and those around us. Bad habits may be pleasant for ourselves, but usually cause annoyance and inconvenience to others.

An efficient business runs smoothly on the good habits of those who work in it. On the other hand, an unsuccessful business does not run smoothly because the habits of those working in it are too slipshod. There is not enough routine. There is not enough co-operation and integration between members of the staff. In other words, a good business is disciplined. A bad business knows no discipline and, because of this, gets nowhere.

We can carry this maxim into our individual lives. If we know where we are going, where we want to go, and make a plan, then we will get there.

Apply this to dieting. We know where we want to go. We want to be slim. We know when we want to go. We want to go now. We want to start right away so that we can reach our goal as soon as possible. In order to do this, then we must conceive a plan. Think again of the good business, the disciplined business. The only way to get there is to make a disciplined plan and stick to it. We must be strict with ourselves. No manager ever made a success of his business unless he was strict with his staff. We must be strict with ourselves, otherwise we will never reach our goal.

Cash in on this habit-forming trait of human nature. Our lives, as we have already noticed, are built up of habits. Some are old, some are not so old and some have been acquired along the way. We are now going to structure our lives so that our habits are very well defined and very well directed. We must think carefully about our eating habits and, if necessary, exchange bad ones for good ones, old ones for new ones.

Sometimes it happens that our whole weight problem was caused in the first place by changing one bad habit for another one. For example, after much struggling we may have managed to stop smoking, but having stopped smoking, something is missing. There is a vacuum in our lives. Nature does not like a vacuum so it tries to fill it. What is easier than to eat a chocolate biscuit with a cup of coffee instead of smoking a cigarette?

Now, it is true that when our body stops receiving the nicotine it has become used to, then our metabolism temporarily slows down. This fact can be used as a convenient excuse for overeating and gaining much weight.

If we stop smoking and leave it at that, then perhaps a pound or two will be gained for a few months, but very quickly our metabolism will readjust itself and these will be lost again. If, on the other hand, knowing that our metabolism is going to slow down, we decide to feed it, then the weight gain will be permanent.

How often do we hear of friends who have stopped smoking and have replaced their cigarette after a meal with a chocolate biscuit? This is what I call the "bending-of-the-elbow" syndrome. We are used to putting something in our mouths as a treat after a good meal. If it can't be a cigarette then a chocolate biscuit will do just as well. People who tend to do this are not really addictive *smokers*, but addictive *"elbow-benders"*. Something has to go into the mouth at regular intervals. What this something is is not terribly important. Such is the force of habit.

As I have already said, habits are formed, or made, and they can be broken. Sometimes performing a certain action can trigger off the thought of food. For example, when you pick up a book, do you automatically think, "Ah, nice and relaxing . . . a cup of coffee with a biscuit"? Or, when dining alone, do you think, "Good, I'm all alone. No need to set the table and make conversation at dinner. I'll just take a tray into the easy chair and eat there." Because you have no company, you pick up a book and start your meal. Your meal goes on and on . . . and on! You are not aware of what you are eating because you are reading. You are just enjoying the sensation of "elbow-bending".

This is a habit that is very easily formed, but can be very hard to break, requiring a great deal of thought and careful planning.

Lone eaters are always at risk. Perhaps because there is not much else to do, or perhaps because they are lonely, they tend to spin out a meal. And what better way to spin out a meal than to eat more of it?

Let us look at what Mrs X is doing.

Mrs X is in a happy, relaxed mood. Her diet has gone well. She has been shopping and has bought a new dress. Just slightly tight, but if she eats a little less she will lose some weight and all will be well.

Arriving home at lunchtime quite hungry after a long morning's shopping, she reviews the situation. Her husband is away on business and the children are at school. Mrs X makes herself a cheese sandwich and a cup of coffee and settles down with a book. The book is very entertaining and Mrs X munches away at her sandwich without being aware of eating it. What she does become aware of, however, is the fact that it is finished, and she's not eating any more.

She glances up from her book and her eyes rest briefly upon a box of chocolates that had been opened the night before. A few minutes later, still reading, she absent-mindedly dips into it and takes a chocolate. She enjoys the pleasant taste of chocolate and, without thinking, takes another. Half an hour later, the chapter is finished — and so are the chocolates! Mrs X looks up in horror and sees what she has done. Another day's dieting spoiled. Oh well, just wait till next Monday and then she'll show the world how it's done!

This incident brings us to another bad habit, that of eating mindlessly. Many people come to visit me in distress about their figures and assure me that they never eat anything. What they actually mean is that they don't eat much at the table, but often, unknown to themselves, they spend their day munching away at a little bit here and a little bit there. This mindless eating can add up to far more than a large meal.

Mindless eaters are quite difficult to deal with because, first of all, they must be convinced that they are eating far more than they are aware of. They just taste the soup to see if it is all right. They have to check if the pudding is lumpy, and the best way to do that is to try a spoonful.

Unfortunately, such mindless tasters tend also to be enthusiastic cooks, so a great deal of their day is spent in the kitchen. Many will tell me that they absorb food through their pores: "I can't possibly become that fat from what I'm eating. The fumes must get to me. The smells must get to me. I never eat what I cook. That is for the family, or for the church, or for the Women's Guild. It's never for me."

That may be so. The food is cooked for others. It's cooked with love and enthusiasm. Unfortunately, however, almost the same amount that is cooked for others is eaten by the cook herself.

It is a physical impossibility to gain weight from the smells and the fumes of cooking. The only way that one can gain weight from cooking is by eating the food. Therefore, these people have first of all to be convinced that they are not absorbing anything except through the mouth.

One of the worst habits, and one which is very common among people with a weight problem, is that of eating in the evening. After work, after the evening meal, once the children are in bed and the washing-up is done, the atmosphere is conducive to relaxation. What better way to relax than staring mindlessly at the television and "bending the elbow"?

One thing that never ceases to surprise me when speaking to such people is their conviction that they are unique in this respect. They come into my consulting-room and are duly given treatment and a diet sheet spiced with good advice. Then, before leaving, they will hesitate and say, "But I have a special problem. My problem is that I start to eat after dinner, and eat steadily through the evening until bedtime."

Most people, I think, would take heart if they knew how often I hear exactly these words. They are ashamed of themselves. They think that there is a great flaw in their characters, that nobody else has this weakness, that everybody else has more will-power and is much stronger and more determined than they are. If they were to just look around them, they would probably find that at least half their family share this weakness; but they don't see it. They feel ashamed and distressed by their inadequacy in dealing with this problem.

There is a well-known proverb which says "A problem shared is a problem halved", and in this case I think it may be true. If people only knew how many other people had the same difficulties, then I think that this would give them the strength and courage they need to try and break this habit.

All habits begin in the brain and therefore all habits must end there. This century has seen a great rise in interest in the workings of that small organ. Great psychologists have sprung up and many have carried out some very interesting experiments, especially in dealing with habits.

It is possible to train animals to do certain things and this training gives us a great insight into our own habits. One experimenter trained rats by giving them food at the sound of a bell. After a while, whenever these rats heard the bell, they produced saliva, knowing they were going to have a meal. After a further period, the experimenter would ring the bell but not give the rats a meal. They had been conditioned and trained to expect food on hearing this bell, and their bodies performed accordingly.

Is this not also a characteristic of human behaviour? How many people on passing a baker's shop and smelling the aroma of freshly baked bread or cakes, will go into that shop and buy? Again, how many people passing a beautifully decorated confectioner's window will not also go into the shop and buy? Are these people hungry? No, of course they are not. They have been conditioned by smell and by sight to anticipate treats.

Again, describe a recipe to a friend. Describe how it is made, how it smells, how it tastes, and that friend will say, "Oh, my mouth is watering." This is another example of conditioning.

Imagination plays a great part in this process. While thinking about food and hearing about how it is prepared, it is possible to imagine that food being prepared and to imagine oneself sitting down to eat it. The body will respond by producing saliva and a feeling of appetite.

Think of the three wise monkeys: "See no evil, hear no evil, speak no evil". We can condition ourselves by sight or sound to expect food. This is a habit.

Sit down and have a good think. What triggers off a sense of appetite in your particular case? Perhaps it is all of these things or perhaps none of them, but there is always something which has this effect in people with a weight problem. If you can isolate what this is or what they are — because some people have many triggers — then you can take steps to deal with them. The habit which causes this urge to eat can thus be broken.

The easiest way to change a habit is to break your routine. Remember, I have said that we are creatures of habit. We like a routine. If we do not follow a routine, then we become disorientated and nothing falls into place. Sit down in the evening in front of the television and, automatically, the "elbow bends". Don't sit down in the evening in front of the television and then disorientation sets in. We don't know what to do. Something has to be found.

This is one of the easiest ways to break a habit. Just change your pattern of living. Instead of sitting down to watch television, do something else. Join a keep-fit class, sew, knit, do a crossword puzzle, anything but watch television, and then your body will be out of co-ordination; the elbow will not automatically bend.

If you know that when you pass a baker's on the way to work in the morning you are going to smell the baking, see if you can find another route to work. If in the evening you know that you are going to pass a confectioner's shop and that you are feeling slightly hungry, your will-power will be at its lowest ebb. See if you can avoid the temptation by taking another route home. Again, if you have a friend who is an enthusiastic cook and who insists on drawing graphic pictures of what she has been cooking, try and talk about something else when you meet her, then you will not rush home to try it for yourself.

Start to follow a whole new lifestyle at the times you find it difficult to do anything but eat. It takes a week or two to break a habit completely. If you think about it, that is not a long time. The first few days are the worst, but each day gets easier. Try not to replace your bad habit by another equally bad habit. Be positive: do something constructive and you will find that you will be much more satisfied within yourself for having broken what might have been a life-long habit.

6

Reasons for Lack of Success

WE HAVE ALREADY spoken about the reasons for being overweight in the first place. These same reasons can also be the cause of lack of success in dieting. They are important enough to talk about again, only this time we will look at them from a different angle. Seen in another setting and from another viewpoint, they will tend to take on a different meaning.

It has crossed the mind of nearly every dieter I know that the reason for not losing weight is physiological in nature rather than psychological. If one's body won't function because of an illness, there is no stigma attached. It just cannot be helped; the dieter is merely the victim of circumstances. On the other hand, any suggestion of psychological involvement can be taken as an insult. People are very loath to admit that their problem is in the mind. Unfortunately, with 99 out of 100 dieters, this is exactly where the problem lies.

There are all sorts of reasons why people fail to have success with their dieting. Some of them are extremely obscure; some are quite simple. Some people read about a diet, feel very enthusiastic about it, and then manage to convince themselves that they are sticking to it without even getting out of the chair. This is not so ludicrous as it sounds. Think about it yourself.

How often have you read some good advice or have read about a diet that attracts you and thought to yourself, "Hey, that's great. That certainly will get the weight off", but have not done anything about it? Wishing will not get you there. It is the practical people who achieve success. The dreamers do not.

Have you ever caught yourself reading a slimming magazine and tucking into a chocolate biscuit at the same time? People who do this are the dreamers. They are the people who will never be successful unless they sit down, have a good think about themselves and get on with it. We have all heard the expression "think positively". Positive thinking will get you there, provided it is followed up by action.

When I was young we had a neighbour who was a strong believer in that whatever you wanted to happen would happen. She did not believe in birth control because her theory was that if you wanted a child you would get one; if you didn't want one, then nothing would happen. Unfortunately, the poor lady ended up with a long string of unplanned children.

Now, this is a good example of wishful thinking. This lady ended up with far more children than she had planned because she did not follow up her positive thinking by positive planning. We can apply the same principle to dieting. We can wish to lose weight and if our desire is strong enough it will be of considerable help along the way, but unless it is backed up by good solid action, then it will not progress beyond the wishing stage and we will get more and more obese and wonder why.

If you have difficulty in losing weight and are convinced that the cause of this is glandular, then your best course of action is to go to your doctor. Explain your problem, and the doctor will do various tests to ensure that your glandular system, like most people's, is in good working order. Having ruled out your glands as an excuse for not losing weight, then you will have to go back to the drawing board and do some serious thinking.

Self-delusion has already been mentioned. As I have said, wishing and believing you can lose weight, or reading about it, are not enough to get you there.

Another reason for failing to lose weight is carelessness when counting calories. This has already been touched upon, but it is crucial to understand that it is very, very important that the calories are carefully counted if you are on a calorie-controlled diet. The only way to count calories is to measure the food first. If this is not done, then your exercise in mental arithmetic is all in vain. In fact, what you are practising is another form of self-delusion. You can delude yourself that you are having 60 calories worth of bread, but in actual fact if you cut a nice thick slice of bread you could be having 120 or 130 calories and still think you're eating 60 calories, because you have learned that one slice of bread contains approximately 60 calories.

I continually reiterate in my clinic that unless the food is measured there will not be much weight loss. Your eye is a very good judge. Unless you are eating junk, your eye sees what the body needs to keep it at the weight it is at the moment. So, if you are given a diet sheet and then ignore the amounts of food that you are allowed on it, then you will find to your great consternation that you look good, you feel good, but, alas, your weight remains static.

Procrastination is another and one of the most common reasons why people do not lose weight. Imagine that you have a stone to lose. You have read in all sorts of magazines and papers that with this, that or the other fabulous diet you can lose a stone in two weeks. So, your thinking goes like this: "I'm a stone overweight, but there's no need to panic because I can lose it in two weeks."

Unfortunately, one stone has a habit of becoming two stones within a very short period of time. Then you think: "Well, if I can lose a stone in two weeks, then I can lose two stones in a month."

It doesn't work like that. These diets in which a large weight loss is achieved in a very short time have the unfortunate side-effect of starving the body of everything it needs. As a consequence, when the diet is no longer adhered to the poor dieter eats everything within sight and the stone lost is very quickly regained — and not only the stone originally lost, but some more besides. Usually, when people lose a stone very quickly, a stone and a half is regained.

This pendulum effect of losing and gaining weight is a cause of great distress to many people. It is better not to lose weight at all and to concentrate on staying the same weight as you are now than to constantly yo-yo up and down, because each loss and gain will see you starting your next diet at a higher weight. Take Mrs X for example:

Mrs X is very excited because she has just read about this fabulous new diet in her magazine. Full of enthusiasm, she goes out to the shops and buys tomatoes, lettuce and a few eggs. These are intended to keep her for a week.

The first day goes well. She is very euphoric, so she has no difficulty in sticking to her diet and is delighted the next morning by a weight loss of two pounds. As the day goes on, she finds herself irritable and disgruntled, but manages to struggle through day two. Again, delight is her emotion the next morning when she finds she has lost a further pound. Great, three pounds in two days!

Day three is even more difficult because, in addition to the irritability that she has been experiencing, she finds that she is a little light-headed, absent-minded and disorientated. She struggles on until lunchtime and then succumbs, not to a nice juicy steak which would have done her little harm, but to the biscuit tin. The dam having been broken, I scarcely need to tell you the end of the story!

Day four sees Mrs X on the scales again. Alas, the three pounds that she has taken off have been regained, but the binge that she has started is not yet satisfied. When Mrs X weighs herself on day five, she finds that she has gained yet another pound. At the end of the week, yet again another pound has gone on. So, when you review Mrs X's fabulous diet, you will find that at the end of the week Mrs X is two pounds heavier than when she started!

Now Mrs X's experience is a very common phenomenon. Most dieters are at some time tempted by the sudden weight loss, although previous experience should have taught them that the gain which follows this will be just as sudden and even more than the loss.

People usually start by thinking: "This time I'll lose a few pounds and then I'll go on a sensible diet and keep it off." The body, however, is very strong. When the resulting lack of various vitamins, minerals and trace elements becomes apparent in the body, then will-power is pushed out the door. The body demands nourishment and nourishment it will get in great amounts to make up for the losses of the previous few days.

Many people who come to me will tell me even before I weigh them that they couldn't possibly have lost weight this week because they have been out. On questioning them further, I find that they have been out one evening. What is one evening consisting of a few hours, out of seven days each consisting of twenty-four hours?

Never consider social eating as an excuse for not having lost weight. One can eat socially and yet manage over the period of a week to get weight off. I think that most people will agree that one of the greatest social eaters that we have ever heard of is our own Queen. If one looks at photographs of the Queen when she was a young woman, she was really quite buxom; then she went on a diet. Having lost weight, despite her busy social life, she has managed, over twenty-five to thirty years, to keep that weight off, which just goes to prove that social eating is an unconvincing excuse for being overweight.

I always divide social eating into three categories: there is the social eating that one does for business (social lunches); there are social evenings spent in friends' homes; and social evenings spent in hotels.

Of these three types the most difficult is the one where one is invited to a friend's home. My advice here is don't be a diet bore. You have been invited to your friend's house and your friend has gone to considerable trouble to entertain you, probably spending the whole day in the kitchen. Then, to be confronted by somebody who says "I'm on a diet. I can't eat any of that" is disheartening, even somewhat insulting.

However, this need not be the case. Usually before dinner at a friend's home, one is offered something to drink; then of course there are the usual side dishes with all sorts of dainty bites on them. However, as long as your glass is full, nobody is going to ask you to have another drink. So, when you take your drink, don't consume it right away; keep your glass full and then nobody can refill it for you. Don't touch what is on the tables. Nobody is going to notice if you are not nibbling nuts. As long as you look as if you are, as long as your glass is full, then nobody will notice and no questions will be asked.

The same applies when you are at the dinner table. There are some foods which you do not have to eat and which will offend nobody if you leave, like a great helping of potatoes or second helpings. Take a little of everything, then say that it was delicious but that you have had quite enough and you don't want to spoil the taste of what you have already eaten by overloading your stomach. The same goes for table wine as it does for the aperitif: keep your glass full, then it will not be topped up.

A social evening in a hotel is much easier. You are paying for the meal, or your host is, therefore you can order what you like. Most hotels have a wide choice of menu and nearly all of them offer at least one dish in every course which is low in calories. If you order this dish, then you will not do yourself too much harm. The same rule applies for drinking wine in an hotel as in a friend's home: don't let your glass become empty, then nobody can fill it up for you.

Many dieters complain bitterly about business lunches. They maintain that their weight comes from eating out every day in a hotel. This should really not be a problem because most hotels offer a salad lunch. Take your car with you and order Perrier water, the excuse for not drinking wine being that you will have to drive.

Social lunches are no excuse whatsoever for being overweight. It is true that you cannot weigh your food as you would at home, but if you stick to salads and avoid alcohol, then little harm will be done.

Alcohol is another common reason for lack of success in dieting. Many people are more than willing to stick to their diet, to weigh every bite they eat, but they are less willing to forego all alcohol. This seems to be very important to them. Let me tell you what alcohol does to the system.

Very often, it is not the high number of calories in a drink that do the damage, but the fact that it contains alcohol. Calories do not count here. The body sees alcohol as a poison which must be got rid of as quickly as possible. It is treated as an emergency, so the liver has to cope with freeing the system of alcohol before it can turn to freeing the system of all the impurities carried to it in the blood.

So what happens when someone takes a drink before dinner? That drink is interpreted by the body as poison. All other foods that have been consumed are put to one side while this alcohol is being processed by the liver. Where is this food stored? It is stored in the tissues as fat. Now, once food has become fat, a whole chemical process must be undergone to release that fat before it can be worked out of the system by the liver. So, once food is stored as fat, it is not quite so easy to get rid of it. The next time you take that harmless little drink just to pick you up before dinner, remember what it is going to do to your dinner!

A further cause of lack of success in dieting is that the dieter, subconsciously, does not want to lose weight and therefore finds all sorts of ways to cheat herself so that she thinks she is dieting; but in actual fact, she is seeing to it that the fat stays where it is because she does not really want to get rid of it. This may be for various underlying reasons, many of which were discussed earlier in this book (see page 14).

Therefore, you should examine your own motives for losing weight. Do you really want to lose it? This is a question that was asked at the very beginning of the book. Make sure that you really do want to lose it and that there are no subconscious factors keeping you back. Once you are certain that you are not subconsciously sabotaging your diet, then you can continue with confidence.

Finally, we come to every dieter's enemy — *the plateau*. This is a stage reached by nearly all dieters. They are sticking to their diet. They are doing everything that they should, yet that weight just will not budge. This is very undermining to any diet and is very discouraging to the dieter, many of whom think: "Oh, it's not working. I'll just give up."

This is the very last thing you should do. Try to imagine what is happening to your body: you are eating less food than the body needs, therefore fat is being used as a reserve. Where does that fat come from? It comes from the fat cells in your body which are gradually emptying. Nature, having no love of a vacuum, very often replenishes some of these fat cells with water. As water is heavier than fat, this means that the scales will not register a weight loss. Funnily enough, though, most people who have reached a plateau find that although they are not losing weight, they are losing inches. The reason for this is that not all the fat cells fill up with water; some of these empty fat cells will cause a reduction which is evident from the tape measure though not from the scales. Remember, your scales can't think. What the scales measure is a total weight, without distinguishing between fat and fluid. The human body is made up almost totally of fluid, and the scales register this.

When a person is losing weight, the fluid table in the body is very unstable. That is why sometimes, in the first week of a diet one can lose seven or eight pounds, yet by doing exactly the same thing the following week can gain three or four. During the first week much fluid will have been lost, but in the second week, once the body gets used to the diet, the fluid balance is restored.

It is this unstable fluid balance that is really the cause of a plateau. The body is carrying more fluid than is normally the case, but eventually it catches up with itself again and the fluid is got rid of. Suddenly the dieter on the plateau finds that several pounds have been lost, as it were, overnight. Sadly, this does not happen to every dieter who reaches a plateau, for the simple reason that they may become discouraged and therefore careless in sticking to their diet. For them, passing beyond the plateau proves impossible and will continue to be so until the dieter gets right back onto the straight and narrow and follows the diet to the letter, after which, the weight loss will start again. Very often, however, reaching a plateau means the end of a diet for some people.

Remember, the body is a very complicated piece of machinery. It is one of the most complicated chemical factories in existence. If you do what you are supposed to do and forget your body, then its chemistry will catch up with itself and you'll be all right, but if you try to force the body to do something that it is not yet ready to do, then you will become discouraged, and in all probability give up dieting. So, concentrate on your part and let the body concentrate on its part and you will find that, in the end, all will be well.

7

Visualisation

NOTHING HELPS A diet better than a vivid and active imagination. If you can visualise the end result of your dieting, then you will be greatly helped in sticking to it.

Think back to the last time you were slim? How well you felt. How confident you felt. What a joy it was to go shopping for clothes. What fun it was going into a crowded changing-room and not feel self-conscious about all the lumps of fat. Never feeling you had to avoid these shops and buy only from shops that had individual changing-rooms. You could go anywhere and you could try on anything without feeling self-conscious.

Do you remember how you used to look forward to an evening out? Never experiencing that feeling of dread and despair as you go through your wardrobe to see what you could wear. Opening your wardrobe and choosing what you felt like wearing that day was a great joy.

Just keep these thoughts in mind. You were slim once, you are meant to be slim, and although you are no longer slim, that need not be a permanent state of affairs. You can become slim again, provided you work at it.

Perhaps you have never been slim. Don't worry. You can still visualise. Think of somebody that you know who is slim. Imagine how she feels. Imagine the ease with which she conducts her life. You too can be like that. Again, though, you must work at it.

The secret of visualisation is positive thought. Don't feed yourself negative thoughts because this will hold back your weight loss. If you say to yourself, "All right, I remember what it was like to be thin, but, alas, it's just a nostalgic memory. Those days will never come again", then the chances are they won't. If you are not convinced within yourself that you can do a thing, then your hope of actually doing it is greatly diminished.

Imagine the feeling of freedom and agility possessed by those who do not have thighs that rub together, who do not have upper arms that quiver like a jelly, who do not have a spare tyre and large tummy and a big bottom. Just imagine being freed from all these things.

As I said earlier, dreaming on its own will not get you there. Your dreams must be backed up by action; then you will savour success. Take visualisation seriously. Plan it into your daily routine. Create visual aids to help you along the way. Find an old photograph of yourself when you were thin and pin it up by your mirror where you can see it daily. Find a dress that you used to wear that you can no longer get into. Hang it up outside the wardrobe and visualise yourself wearing it — not the *last* time you wore it, but the *next* time!

If you have never been slim and therefore have no photograph of yourself, then cut one out of a magazine of somebody you admire, somebody who has a figure that is pleasing to you. Imagine that you are that person. Keep looking at it and keep telling yourself that if you work at it, you can be like that too.

The power of visualisation was recognised by an unknown American chemist about fifty years ago. Every time he handed his customers a prescription, he would also give them the advice to say to themselves two or three times a day, "Every day in every way, I am becoming a little better". People who did this discovered that, indeed, every day in every way they did become a little better. This is because this saying had penetrated into their subconscious mind, which in turn started to work for them and to help them to improve.

We, too, can use our subconscious minds in order to help us to lose weight, but first of all, let us have a look at that subconscious mind. This is the part of the brain that stores knowledge. Everything that we learn goes in there. It can be programmed like a computer. In fact, it acts just like a computer, and also like a computer has no conscience or judgement. Everything that we know or have learned is stored there and can be very easily recalled or relearned. All we have to do is think about it and it will float up to the conscious mind, where it can be used.

The subconscious mind will obey the conscious mind; any command given to it will be obeyed. We can use this to our advantage if we want to slim, but we must first know how to reach the subconscious mind. There are several layers of subconscious, but the one we want to reach is very near the surface and is easily accessible with a little bit of practice.

The first step is to think carefully about what you want to tell your subconscious mind. Don't make it too complicated; just a few short commands. Having made up your mind what you want to imprint on your subconscious mind, then you will need to get into it. The easiest way to do this is by relaxing. You can do this either sitting or lying down. If you are sitting, find a chair that is comfortable. Do not cross your arms or legs. Just sit with your feet together and your hands on your lap or on the arms of the chair.

All around us there is a great energetic force called the *life-force*. Here, we would like to tap into this because it will strengthen us. In order to do this, lie or sit with your palms facing upwards and your thumb and your middle finger joined to form a circle. This will draw the life-force around you towards yourself and give you power.

Another great source of energy lies within ourselves, and we have easy access to that as well. Instead of holding your palms face upwards to face the cosmos, put your left hand on your stomach at a point just below your navel and place your right hand on top of it. This will balance the life-force within you and also give you extra power. Use whichever of these two methods you find the easiest or most relaxing.

Having got yourself comfortable, then concentrate on relaxing individual parts of your body. Start at your toes and work up over your feet and legs, up through your body, down through your arms, and up again into your neck and head. Every single part of your body must be relaxed.

While you are doing this, breathe for relaxation. Think about your breath as the oxygen in the air and imagine that you are taking it into yourself and into the fibres of your body, as a great source of extra energy. Think of your body as being completely hollow, to be filled with great breaths of oxygen. In order to do this properly, breathe in through your nose and down into your stomach cavity. From there, feel the air going right down through all your limbs and then hold your breath for a few seconds before letting it out slowly through your open mouth.

Repeat this exercise five or six times. While you are doing it, keep your eyes open at a point just slightly above eye-level. When your eyes begin to feel heavy, let them fall shut.

Complete relaxation takes some practice, but it doesn't matter if you don't get it right the first time. When you feel you have got as relaxed as you can that is the time to start suggesting to your subconscious mind what you want it to learn; perhaps you might suggest to it just a simple statement: "I don't like sweets", for example.

Repeat this two or three times, all the while breathing steadily in as relaxed a position as possible. After you have said this a few times, start imagining yourself as slim. Think of yourself in a setting that you enjoy, for example, in a sunny garden. Imagine yourself walking around that garden. You are slim. You can feel the movement of your limbs , the agility that you have, the ease with which you walk, unencumbered by the rolls of fat. Let this pleasant thought linger in your mind for a little while and then stretch slowly, open your eyes and lie or sit still for a few seconds. You will find that you will be in a very relaxed, refreshed frame of mind.

Repeat this whole exercise once or twice per day and in a surprisingly short period of time it will take effect. Good times to do it are on waking up in the morning and just before going to sleep at night.

Gradually feed more information to your subconscious mind. Don't overload it; one command or one suggestion at a time is enough, otherwise confusion sets in. It has been found that it works better if it is done gradually. Suggest one thing, and then when you feel that you have mastered that, suggest the next phase; then gradually work up until you are completely conditioned and set up for success.

Remember that you also have the help of your visual aids. Keep looking at your slim photograph or your slim picture. Keep looking at the dress that you couldn't get into. Try it on occasionally and see if there is a difference.

Keep this slim image of yourself in your mind constantly. Many dieters become discouraged because they have a fat image of themselves. Long after they have lost their weight they still carry around in their head this fat image of themselves and they find it extremely difficult to realise that they have actually lost the weight and are now slim. In some cases it takes almost a year for the mental image of oneself to catch up with the actual image. If you visualised yourself as being slim right from the start, then this will not be necessary.

Many people who have retained a fat image of themselves after becoming slim have overdone things and even gone as far as to become anorexic. So, right at the very beginning, make sure that your image of yourself is a slim one. What you are seeing in the mirror is not what you are going to see in a very few short months. So, make sure you are ready for it. This is a very positive action because this imagery helps us to reach our goal much more quickly.

As I have already said, your subconscious mind will obey your conscious one. Some people find the method I have described above to be very successful for spot reducing. If one has too large a bosom, if one can imagine oneself with a small bosom, then the subconscious will get to work and help to achieve this.

Regular practice is necessary,' but the stronger you believe in the power of positive thought, then the better it will work for you. So, start practising now, and while you are sticking to your diet, you will find that this will make it so much easier. Steer clear of negative thoughts, because negative thoughts lead to negative actions. The more positive you can be, the better you are going to set yourself up for success, the easier you are going to be able to follow your diet, and the sooner you are going to attain the figure in the photograph.

8

Dietary Aids

MANY PEOPLE FIND it difficult to stick to a diet unless they have some help. That help can either come in human form, in the form of treatment, or in the form of pills.

For some people, losing weight proves to be impossible without the help and encouragement of an adviser. The responsibility of having to answer for their actions to a stranger is enough to make them stick to their diet, apart from the fact that they are ashamed of standing on the scales and being found to weigh the same or even more than they did the week before.

These are the easiest people to deal with. Others have much more need of counselling. It is necessary to get to the root of their troubles and to talk it out with them. Many people respond well to group therapy; for this purpose a large number of popular clubs have sprung up where people can come together to be weighed by an adviser, after which a lecture is given and ideas are exchanged between members.

Although this approach is very successful for a great many people, there are others who find that this represents an encroachment on their privacy. Such people find it much easier to communicate on a one-to-one basis. Since this book has so far dealt solely with this type of communication, I will not embroider further upon it.

Next we come to the treatment of obesity. Several forms of treatment are known and commonly used and have proved very popular. These are hypnotherapy, acupuncture or acupressure, slimming pills and exercise.

Although some people are enthusiastic about hypnotherapy, we do not use this method in our clinic because I find that imposing one's will upon another's half-conscious mind can sometimes lead to complications. Some people who are extremely sensitive can react badly to this method and so we avoid it.

The most successful method that I have found till now is the use of acu-aids. This involves a harmless procedure which balances the body and makes it much easier for the hypothalamus to work, ensuring a weight loss. The hypothalamus is a small gland in the brain and has been called the pleasure centre of the mind.

I have already mentioned that a baby cannot be forced to eat more than it needs. The reason for this is that, at this age, the hypothalamus is in good working order. As we get older, this gland, through various bad habits, ceases to function as it should. It really acts as a sort of appetite conscience, and like the ordinary conscience it functions accordingly. If we ignore our conscience often enough, then it ceases to function. The same goes for the hypothalamus. If we constantly ignore the warnings that we have had enough to eat then the hypothalamus will eventually cease to tell us that we are full. We can eat mindlessly, with nothing, no "conscience", to stop us.

Using acupressure, we can reactivate this function of the hypothalamus, so that we become much more aware and much more willing to stop eating when we have had enough.

Along with the acu-aid treatment, I also prescribe herbal slimming pills. These are designed to suppress the appetite so that no hunger pangs are experienced. This, along with a sensible diet, usually does the trick.

I find it difficult to make some people understand that slimming pills in themselves will not make them slim. All a slimming pill will do is suppress the appetite so that one is less inclined to eat more than one should. Nevertheless, if a diet is not adhered to, then any number of slimming pills will be useless.

Extensive research has gone into the development and manufacture of slimming pills. The drug companies now have quite a variety, working on various principles, on the market. Many of these pills, although they do suppress the appetite, can be very dangerous in other ways in that they can cause unpleasant side-effects.

Although these anti-obesity drugs help weight loss, like their herbal counterparts they do so only in conjunction with a diet. Again, they are not magic. A diet has to be adhered to, otherwise everything will be in vain.

The least dangerous of these pills are the type known as bulking agents. These are made of a substance called methyl cellulose and act by swelling up in the stomach when taken with water, helping to prevent a feeling of hunger. These can be very useful for people who are genuinely hungry, but those who are addictive eaters receive little benefit because even when such people are full, they will still want to eat.

Another type of drug is the central nervous system stimulant. These drugs can have very nasty side-effects in that they cause an initial feeling of euphoria, which makes it extremely easy to become addicted to them. This is the reason why many doctors are reluctant to prescribe these drugs. When they are prescribed, it is generally only on a short-term basis.

We get a very different picture when we talk about herbal slimming pills. These pills are non-addictive, have few or no side-effects, and are completely harmless.

At the moment I am in the process of developing a new slimming aid which will be manufactured in

Switzerland by Bioforce and will soon be available on the open market. It is designed to suppress the appetite and speed up the body metabolism. It also contains a mild diuretic in the form of the Jerusalem artichoke, which is one of nature's most effective fluid eliminators. To my mind, no slimming aid has ever been so successful. It is completely without danger and contains no artificial preservatives, colourings, or other additives. Even without an accompanying diet, this remedy will certainly help to suppress the appetite, although if substantial weight losses are to be achieved, a diet still must be adhered to.

In addition to its other virtues, this preparation helps to strengthen the nervous system, so that those who find difficulty in dieting because of worry or stress will find that they feel much calmer and thus more able to concentrate on a diet.

As I said earlier, most people have a glandular system which is in perfect working order. However, one or two per cent of the population do suffer from glandular malfunction. There are people who eat a lot and remain extraordinarily thin, and others who eat very little food and still put on weight. Everything, they say, turns to fat.

Progressive research has shown that dysfunction of the glands which discharge their hormones directly into the bloodstream can be partially responsible for both excessive corpulence or excessive thinness. The glands primarily responsible for this are the pituitary, the ovaries, the testicles and the thyroid. Over-function or imbalance usually leads to thinness, while sub-function of any of them leads to corpulence.

It has been observed that the removal of the ovaries or a disease that leads to their sub-functioning often causes a person to put on weight. The frequent incidence of women gaining weight after the change of life would tend to confirm this fact. A typical example can be seen if we consider inhabitants of a southern climate: people who live in Italy or South America are usually very slim when they are young; as soon as they approach the change of life, usually at a much earlier age than in temperate climates, the glandular secretions diminish and they become plump.

If the problem is ovarian, then it is quite easily dealt with. A treatment called Sitzbaths stimulates the ovaries and is of immense help in reducing corpulence. Pituitary obesity is not so easy to deal with, because this gland is less amenable to corrective treatment than the ovaries. There are, of course, glandular preparations on the market which do act on the pituitary, but, as with all other similar remedies, their administration is a delicate undertaking. Furthermore, these preparations do not always produce positive results.

The ovaries, as previously mentioned, are much more easily treated by special preparations on the market. However, the simplest expedient that can be recommended, which will stimulate the functioning of the ovaries, is to consume various foods that contain vitamin E. The most important of these is wheatgerm. There are people who won't eat wheatgerm for fear of getting fat, because it has also been recommended to thin people who wish to gain weight. Women need not worry about this, for wheatgerm and its vitamin E content only regulate the function of the ovaries, stimulating their function in the case of fat people, and reducing their function in the case of thin people. Apart from vitamin E it also contains other valuable nutrients like protein, phosphates and natural sugar. All these have a beneficial effect on the body without any danger of an abnormal weight gain. Thus, anybody suffering from obesity should not hesitate to take wheatgerm, for it will not increase weight, but oppose it.

Natural vitamins also help to regulate the body's working. Synthetic vitamins can be dangerous if too large a dose is taken. With natural vitamins, the situation is different. If too many are taken, the body will eliminate the excess, thus making them quite safe for everyday use. If you feel that you could benefit from a course of vitamins, make sure that you know the source of these vitamins, so that you are taking the ones that help you, without damaging your health.

Sometimes the source of our excess weight can lie in the gonads. If such functional abnormalities have been existing since youth, the gonad glands will generally be found to be underdeveloped, or at least inactive, with no hormonal production. Often in such cases, fat is deposited on the hips and waist only, and never on the extremities. In women, the breasts show a considerable fat deposit, instead of being made up of well-developed milk-producing glands.

Sagging breasts are often an additional worry of overweight women. This problem can be related to the malfunctioning of the ovaries. This type of obesity cannot be dealt with by means of special diets or any other kind of treatment. It can be overcome only if the causes of it are treated. This means a stimulation of the production of the gonads, the thyroid and the pituitary.

When choosing remedies we will certainly want to turn to marine plants such as kelp preparations, which are of excellent value. Bee pollen will be of additional help, since it is known to have stimulating effects.

In order to take full advantage of the various foods available on our diet, we should drink plenty of beet, carrot and celery juices. Young stinging nettles or grated horseradish should also be eaten daily. As a supplement to our diet, oysters, shrimps and octopus have great therapeutic value. Extracts from animal glands may also be helpful, but only if taken in the appropriate dosages; otherwise they may do more harm than good. In addition, exercise — walking, hiking and jogging — and deep breathing, preferably in mountain or sea air, are excellent for stimulating the glands.

One product which we rarely see nowadays is excellent for dealing with obesity. This is whey concentrate. Milk has always been regarded as a remedial food and whey has also been applied externally in the form of packs to alleviate complaints such as inflammation of the gall bladder. While curd packs are also well known, whey, which constitutes the serum of the milk, is the remedy used most often. Whey contains most of the mineral nutrients we require, while cheese, from whose manufacture whey is derived, is valued chiefly on account of its high protein and fat content. The rennet used to make cheese doubtlessly plays an important part in the therapeutic effects of the whey.

Milk itself is a wholefood, which implies that it contains all the necessary elements to sustain life. Among these elements are proteins, carbohydrates, fats, minerals, vitamins and trace elements. Since cheese chiefly contains the proteins and fat present in milk, whey, the by-product of its manufacture, still has considerable nutritional value. It is therefore of little wonder that in former times royalty and the famous from France and other countries made special journeys to Switzerland to take the world-renowned Swiss whey cure. Usually, the visitors were afflicted with metabolic problems such as obesity, circulatory congestions, intestinal ills, pancreatic deficiencies and so on, although whey cures were prescribed for a multitude of other conditions as well.

The benefits of whey concentrate are many. Digestion can be greatly assisted if a tablespoonful or even a teaspoonful of whey concentrate is added to a glass of mineral or ordinary water. Whey concentrate appears to regulate the secretion of gastric acid, for it reduces an excess of acid and increases its quality. When there is a lack of acid, it also benefits diabetes, because the lactic ferments stimulate the pancreas. Thus, it is without a doubt one of the best drinks most patients could wish for.

The regular use of whey concentrate will lower the blood-sugar level and, at the same time, reduce the quantity of sugar in the urine. The results will not be experienced overnight; it will take several weeks for these effects to manifest themselves, but with patience and persistence a positive change for the better will be realised.

The products I have mentioned so far are manufactured by Dr Vogel, under the trade name of Bioforce. The whey concentrate is marketed under the name of Molkosan. The kelp product is called Kelpasan and the slimming drops are called Bio-slim. Ovarisan will stimulate the ovaries. These products are readily available in most health food shops, but should you find difficulty in procuring some item that you would like to try, the address and telephone number from which they can be obtained are provided in the list at the end of the book.

Another company which produces good supplements for slimmers is Nature's Best. One product I would like to mention here is L-Carnitine. Carnitine is an amino acid which plays an important role in fat metabolism and is essentially for the transport of fatty acids into the mitochondria matrix. Research into the way our bodies use this nutrient has shown that the energy released when fat metabolism takes place may help to maintain the stamina required during strenuous exercise.

Carnitine is made in the liver from lysine, with the help of vitamin C, the B vitamins and iron. Virtually no carnitine is available in vegetables; the main sources are red meat and dairy foods. Strict vegetarians therefore need to synthesise their own carnitine from lysine.

Another very active product from Nature's Best is W and A Control. This is made up of four amino acids and vitamins C, B_1, B_6 and B_7 and has proved very beneficial to people following a weight loss programme, although it is not recommended for those suffering from hypertension or phenyketonuria. Two of the best supplements, also from Nature's Best, are the G H R Daytime and Night Time formulas. These contain a high potency of amino acids and vitamins, providing nutrients and helping the process of fat metabolism and the maintenance of muscle tone, even while you are sleeping.

G H R Daytime formula is certainly different from G H R Night Time because each nutrient in both is selected to take account of the body's bio-rhythms. Both, however, contain L-ornithine. This is a substance that is very active in the body when people are young, but by the age of 25/30, it becomes almost non-existent. It is the growth hormone responsible for helping children to grow healthily. It regulates the metabolism, causing a child to grow, rather than to become fat, and is at its most active after strenuous physical exercise or during sleep. In an adult, this substance will stimulate muscle growth but not fat production; therefore, if it is taken as a supplement, a person will become less flabby and more firm and will have a better contoured body.

Because Nature's Best has developed these supplements on a homoeopathic basis, they are completely safe to take. Like Dr Vogel's remedies, Nature's Best remedies can be obtained in most health food shops. Again, should you find difficulty in obtaining them, the address of the company is provided at the end of this book.

You will remember that I have said that very few people have true difficulties with their glands. The chances are that if you were truly suffering from a hormonal or glandular problem then it would already have been diagnosed by your doctor.

The products described above will stimulate the body. They will stimulate your glands and hormones, but they will not necessarily cure any dysfunction. You will, however, by using these products, experience a sense of well-being that you have perhaps never felt before. Remember, though, that only in conjunction with a diet will these products work for you. They only help. It is your diet, yourself, your own frame of mind that does the work of slimming your body.

9

Exercise

THERE IS NO end to the forms of exercise that can serve their purpose in a slimming programme. For many people who decide to take up a regular exercise programme, slimming seems to be their main objective.

Exercise can be very helpful in speeding up weight loss. What happens when you exercise is that you speed up your metabolism. In other words, you make your fat burn more quickly. So, if two people were to follow the same diet and one exercised and the other didn't, the chances are that the active person would experience a better and quicker weight loss than the inactive one, a further bonus being that the active person would develop smooth, supple muscles, whereas for the inactive person, although the weight would come off, the body would stay flabby.

Remember, however, that by incorporating exercise into a slimming programme one's general fitness will also benefit greatly. When your muscles are toned up, your physical appearance will immediately improve.

I have often noticed that the New Year is seen as a turning point for many, when people make up their minds to undo some of the damage caused by over-indulgence over the previous few weeks. Simply cutting down their food intake will obviously result in some weight loss. If the problem is merely a few pounds gained over the previous few weeks, there is little to worry about as this is quickly and easily rectified. However, if it concerns excess weight that has been carried for a longer period, then it is advisable to combine dietary efforts with a programme of exercise in order to obtain a higher degree of fitness as well as weight reduction.

Only by developing a feeling of physical and mental well-being can we look and feel good. Exercise can stimulate the body in a way that nothing else can. It can give you a feeling of vigour and well-being that far exceeds your greatest expectations. However, exercise must always be treated with respect and must be embarked upon gradually. Do not suddenly decide that you are going to start leading a very active life. This is very dangerous. If in the past you have found it a great effort even to walk as far as your car, then don't think that you will be able to jog a mile. Don't even attempt it. It could be fatal!

Most of us start out with good intentions, but within a short period these good intentions tend to diminish. The time needed for a few exercises is not excessive, but keeping it up requires a measure of mental and physical discipline. Too often exercise is put off till tomorrow because something has cropped up or we just are not in the right mood. Mental sluggishness can be overcome by physical exercise and this is a benefit that is often overlooked.

Not all people actually get enjoyment out of regular exercise such as walking, jogging, swimming or cycling, and especially if they do not have a weight problem this is placed low on their list of priorities. However, as I have said before, physical well-being goes hand-in-hand with mental well-being and alertness.

In this chapter I intend to place the accent on an exercise plan that is combined with a slimming programme. I will first describe a number of exercises designed to work on specific parts or functions of the body and will then proceed to discuss a sensible approach to other forms of exercise.

First and foremost, however, please remember the importance of posture and never allow yourself to slouch. Always stand, sit or walk tall. Straighten the back, pull in the stomach and stretch the neck! Any lifting at all should be done with a straight spine and bent knees, while any effort should come from the legs and not the back. This is what is meant when the expression "vertical lifting" is used. The following simple hints will ensure correct posture:

—Point your toes straight forward when walking.
—Place most of your weight on the heels.
—Place your chest forward and elevate the front of the pelvis as if walking up an incline.
—Avoid wearing high heels.
—Stand as if you are trying to touch the ceiling with the top of your head and direct your eyes straight ahead.

Breathing exercises can also be very beneficial. Train yourself to breathe properly. Practise breathing exercises in the fresh air by standing tall and breathing in through the nose. Slowly count up to five holding your breath and pulling in the stomach. Count to five again and then exhale with your mouth wide open, expelling all the air. Relax and repeat six times to begin with, gradually increasing to fifteen times.

Please also remember that exercises need not be strenuous to be effective; nevertheless, always concentrate on the muscles you are using.

Stomach exercises

These exercises largely concentrate on the stomach muscles and it is best if they are done first thing in the morning.

—Stand in a relaxed manner in the correct posture, i.e. with a straight back. Then tense your stomach muscles as if preparing to receive a blow. Pull in the stomach muscles as tightly as possible and maintain the tension while

slowly counting to ten before releasing.
Repeat three times.

—Sit on the floor with your feet parallel and knees slightly
bent. Clasp your hands together and then place them at
the back of the neck. Push your elbows back. Keeping
your trunk straight and elbows out to the side, move
your trunk forward and then back.
Do this exercise ten times.

—Sit on the floor with your legs together and toes stretched.
Remember to keep your spine straight. Now stretch your
toes as if trying to touch the floor and after that pull them
back as far as possible towards your body. Feel the
stretches alternately in the front and in the back of the
legs.
Repeat this exercise twelve times.

Hip exercises
Hip exercises are also very much in demand. These are
important not only because they help to reduce the size of
one's hips, but also because they enable one to retain
maximum flexibility in these joints.

—Lie back on the floor with your knees bent and feet apart.
Relax the head and neck. Clasp your hands behind your
knees and bring the knees up to the chest. Take a deep
breath and exhale.
Do this exercise at least ten times.

—Stretch out on the floor and pull up your knees so that
both feet are placed flat on the floor just in front of the
buttocks. Slowly raise your hips and then slowly lower
the spine again back onto the floor.
Rest and repeat ten times.

Arm exercise
—Stand upright with your feet slightly apart and arms
folded across the chest. Place the palms of your hands
against the biceps and slightly lift the elbows. Push for a

count of five.
Repeat four to six times.

Leg exercises
—Stand upright with your feet slightly apart and toes
  pointed outwards. Stretch your arms out to the side and
  bend your knees so that your hips are positioned above
  the knees. Straighten your legs and press back your
  knees.
  Do this exercise at least eight times.

—For this good loosening-up exercise stand alongside a
  piece of furniture and hold on to this for support. When
  using the right hand for support, swing the left leg
  forwards and backwards with your toes pointed. Slightly
  raise your hip so that your foot just brushes over the
  floor. Try to avoid jerking the spine. Change hands and
  repeat with the other leg.
  Swing at least ten to fifteen times with each leg, attempting to progressively increase the height of the swinging
  motion.

—Kneel down and bend your head forward so that it comes
  to rest on your folded arms resting on the floor. Stretch
  and raise your left leg behind your body, keeping your
  toes pointed. Then make small circular movements with
  your foot in both directions, while counting to five.
  Lower your leg and repeat with the other one.
  Complete at least five lifts with each leg to begin with,
  gradually building up to ten.

Back exercise
This exercise is very useful for keeping the spine straight
and flexible.

—Stand flat with your back against a door, touching the
  door with as many parts of the body as possible, e.g.
  heels, calves, buttocks, shoulders and head. Slowly
  bend your knees and slide down, while continuing to
  touch the door with the whole of the upper body.

Straighten your body up again. Do this ten times, if at all possible without using anything for support. Older people and those who suffer from back problems are advised to place a chair in front of them for support.

Yoga exercises
Many yoga exercises are also suitable for gentle toning-up of the muscles. The examples given here are excellent in this respect.

—Sit cross-legged on the floor. Reach up high with your left hand and with a semi-circular movement bring your hand down to the left of your waist. Gently rock sideways as if trying to touch the floor with your hooked elbow. Stretch in the opposite direction and then return to the starting position. You should remember that this exercise should be done slowly and harmoniously, without jerking. Try and make it a flowing movement.
Do this exercise six times, then change arms and repeat on the other side.

—Again sit cross-legged on the floor, with your spine held straight. Look straight ahead and fix your eyes on something stationary. Lean slowly forward from the waist, bringing your head as close to the ground as possible. Then straighten up again.
Repeat this exercise several times.

—Stand upright with your legs slightly apart and back hollowed. Let your arms hang loose beside your body. Bend the upper part of your body forward from the hips and swing your outstretched arms backwards and forwards between the legs.
Slowly do ten swings to begin with and gradually increase this number with practice.

—A variation of this exercise is to hold an object of a certain weight in your hands while doing it. Aim to gradually increase the weight of the object.

—Stand with your legs astride and lean over so that your

arms hang loose. Then gently swing your arms to the side, trying to reach a little further each time. This is the so-called "pendular exercise".
Do this exercise twelve times to begin with, slowly increasing.

—A progression from the pendular exercise is to swing the arms out to the sides and on the third swing the arms are held stretched out for a count of five.
Repeat ten times.

—You can progress further by holding a book or another object in each hand as you do the exercise. As the arms get stronger the weight of these objects can be gradually increased to approximately 2 lbs.

—Place one leg in front of the other, bend over from the waist as before and swing your arms backwards and forwards beside the body. Progress from this by doing three swings and then holding the arms steady for a count of five. Progress yet again by holding weights as you do it.

—Stand with your legs slightly apart and with your arms hanging loose beside your body. Swing your arms out and then in again several times. Then keep your arms stretched out and make circular movements with your hands — six times forwards and six times backwards. Gradually build up the number of movements as the arms get stronger. You can also aim to do this exercise with your arms held at shoulder height.

The best back support is derived from one's own back muscles. Regular back exercises, if done correctly, can often help to avoid the need for an external brace or corset. Back muscles can give the body all the necessary support if they are strengthened by routine performance of the prescribed exercises. If possible, follow the exercise routine prescribed by your own doctor or osteopath. Gradually increase the frequency of the exercises as your condition improves and also increase the amount of exercise, but always stop when you begin to feel tired.

If your arms or legs feel tight, then take a warm shower or bath before performing back exercises. Do not be alarmed if you experience slight discomfort afterwards. This should diminish as the muscles become stronger. Stop doing any exercise that causes pain and if possible check with your practitioner as to the suitability of that particular exercise.

Never overdo your exercises, especially in the early stages of an exercise programme. Try to do all the movements slowly and carefully. Again, do not be afraid if these exercises sometimes cause a mild discomfort which lasts for a few minutes. Do all floor exercises on a hard surface, covered by a thin mat or rug or a heavy blanket. Place a pillow under the neck if it will make you more comfortable or even a thin pillow under the small of the back. Wear loose clothing and remove any footwear. Always follow your practitioner's instructions carefully and it will be well worth the effort.

Exercises can become a pleasurable part of one's life and when combined with sensible dietary management, the toned and firmed-up muscles will become noticeable in a relatively short period of time.

Always visualise yourself as the slim and healthy person you would like to be. Keep in mind your posture, concentrate the mind on it and make the muscles work. The reward will soon be noticeable, not only in your outward appearance, but also in an increased feeling of fitness and health.

As we move on now to other types of excercise I should perhaps add a word of caution for all those who exercise. For the best part of thirty years I have worked in an osteopathic practice, but over the latter few years I have noticed a change in the patients who consult me. Recently I have found all too frequently that slimmers are too enthusiastic and think that with excessive exercise the weight will come off more quickly. Nothing could be further from the truth.

Exercises that are done solely for slimming purposes need to be of low intensity and long duration as this is the only way that the body fat will be reduced. If you enter an exercise programme too enthusiastically, you may still burn up fat, but this could be replaced by muscle tissue. Although men are more prone to this than women, there is no golden rule that this only happens to men, as there are plenty of exceptions to this rule. Always remember that there is nothing common about common sense.

It is especially as a result of aerobics and jogging that many slimmers have turned up in my waiting-room for osteopathic treatment. Jogging and aerobics are really quite strenuous forms of exercise and a reasonable physical condition is necessary before such activities should be embarked upon. If such spare-time activities appeal to you, great care must be taken that a sensible programme is adhered to and that the intensity of this programme is gradually built up along the lines discussed below.

Aerobics

I am not generally in favour of aerobic exercises. Of course, walking, jogging, swimming and cycling are all aerobic, but by aerobic exercises I mean those involving sudden jerks of the body which can strain the muscles or put out the back and cause great pain. Such exercises are harmful and unnecessary. Exercise need not, indeed must not, be painful. Do it gently, enjoy it, feel your muscles working, but don't strain them to the extent of causing pain. Don't stretch further than is comfortable. Don't run longer than you are able.

One good way of exercising at home is just to tape some lively music and dance to it. If necessary, pretend you are very good at it and introduce variety into your dancing. To start with, do this on your own so that you will not be self-conscious and will not be over-exerting yourself. You will find that, gradually, you will be able to do do more, to do it more vigorously, and to do it for longer. But always remember that with this sort of exercise you must warm up beforehand and then cool down afterwards.

Walking and Jogging

I find that walking is one of the best forms of exercise for beginners. Walk on your own, so that you do not have to pace yourself by others. Don't overdo it. When you start, a twenty-minute gentle walk is enough. Each day, try to extend the distance that you walk in the twenty minutes.

Keep this up for two or three weeks. When you have reached the stage that you can walk briskly, let's say at four miles an hour, then you are ready to start jogging gently, but don't do this in one fell swoop. Perhaps you could start by jogging for twenty paces, then walking for twenty paces. Keep this up for twenty minutes, then gradually extend the amount of jogging you do and make the walking periods shorter. In this way, you can build up your ability to jog without harming yourself.

The most important rule for a jogger to remember is to allow them-selves a warm-up period and a cooling-down period. To warm up you can walk briskly until you begin to feel warm; only then should you start jogging. At the end of your jog, slow down to a walking pace and then walk at a normal pace until you have cooled down. This is very important because failing to warm up or cool down could lead to too much strain being placed on the heart and this spells disaster.

Remember also to wear appropriate shoes, as most jogging is done on paved surfaces that are hard underfoot and can cause jerking of the joints or ligaments. Always put the heel down with each step and run tall. Keep the upper body relaxed and the hands loose at the sides and try to be as relaxed as possible while jogging, again bearing in mind that the surface can be very hard.

To finish off an exercise programme it is advisable to do some stretching exercises. This applies to any form of exercise, not only to jogging. Any exercise causes the muscles to thicken and shorten. If they have been worked hard the muscles will then actually bunch up. Often the resulting muscle-ache makes us feel good as we then consider that we have given it our very best. This way, however, we are much more prone to injuries. Therefore slow and gentle stretching of the muscles after a bout of exercise is very important. Do not jerk the muscles but slowly stretch them. For example, place your right hand on a wall slightly above head height and move your left leg backwards, pressing the knee back so that the muscles in the back of the leg are really stretched, as will be the muscles in the right arm. Stretch for approximately one minute and then repeat with the other arm and leg.

Another good stretching exercise is to bend at the knees, resting your hands with the fingertips on the floor in front of the body. Then stretch your right leg sideways away from the body. Rest your heel on the floor and stretch the leg muscles. Gently ease into this position and do not jerk. Repeat this exercise with the other leg.

Swimming

If you elect to go swimming as a means of exercise, then again, go carefully. As with walking, swim alone and set your own pace. Start very gently, perhaps making your target one length of the pool with no particular time to get there. As the days go by, you could then either increase the amount of swimming that you do or shorten the amount of time that you take to swim your length. Again, gradually build this up until you feel that you are covering the distance or taking the time that you would wish in order to give yourself enough exercise.

Cycling

Cycling is another good form of exercise. Again, don't go too far. Don't go up too many hills to start with. Proceed at your own pace. It doesn't matter if everybody else goes faster. You set your own pace and then you gradually extend both your distance and your pace until you are doing quite vigorous exercise. Before taking up cycling it is always wise to check that the height of the saddle is correct so that the legs are almost fully extended on each downwards movement and that the handlebars are adjusted accordingly.

Stationary bicycles or home trainers have lots of added extras. The biggest advantages they possess are that the resistance can be increased to make the legs work harder and both speed and "distance" can be measured. These are valuable points when one intends to build up a serious training programme. However, again a word of warning is required. Always warm up slowly and never jump into the saddle and start pedalling away frantically. Pace yourself and gradually push yourself to either a higher speed or more effort. The main disadvantage of home trainers is that the exercise does not take place in the fresh air.

There are of course many more forms of exercise that are of great help to slimmers, such as rowing, skipping, and many other sporting activities. Whichever appeals to you, never forget that the golden rule is to always warm up properly and always check your breathing. Remember that any form of exercise affects the rate of your heartbeat.

Having read this chapter and the one which precedes it, you will now realise that there are many other things apart from dieting that can help you on your way to being an attractive person.

It was said earlier in the book that the scales cannot think; they can merely record a person's weight — and a person's weight is made up of many things. Moreover, it is not just your weight that will make you slim. It is the way in which you stand. It is the way in which you walk. The way that you feel. These things cannot be recorded on the scales.

Remember, if you have been exercising and have worked up some fine muscles, that muscle weighs more than fat and you may not be as light on the scales as you would like to be. But look at yourself and measure yourself. You will find that you have a much more attractive figure, and, on the whole, because of your new lifestyle, are a much more attractive person.

10

The Hare and the Tortoise

WHEN WE START a new diet, our main aim is to lose as much weight in as short a time as possible. Usually this aim is realised in the first week of a new diet, because as well as losing fat we tend to lose a lot of water.

Unfortunately, week two can see a very different pattern. Perhaps just one pound will be lost and as a result we feel disappointed. There is no need to feel discouraged, because week two will also have seen a regain of some of that lost fluid. So, in fact, it is more than one pound of fat that has been lost in week two. It is just that the scales only register one pound.

Week three will perhaps see a greater weight loss, because the body will by then be balanced and not much fluid will be lost. The weight loss will be fat alone. Thereafter, if you persevere, you will find that with a good slimming diet your weight should settle down to a weight loss of about two to three pounds a week, which is as much as the human body can afford to lose and yet still continue to feel well and function as it should. Unfortunately, many people are too impatient. They want a bigger weight loss in a shorter time and so they turn to crash diets.

If this is what you want to do, there is no shortage of synthetic crash diets on the market. The last few years has seen the birth of what are known as the very low-calorie diets, the most famous of which is, of course, the "Cambridge Diet".

These diets claim to provide all the vitamins, minerals and trace elements that a person needs every day. This is true. What the advertising for these diets does not say is that they are starvation diets; the body reacts as if it were being starved. The first thing that happens is that the metabolism slows down, even, in rare cases, shuts down altogether. The body is in a crisis. It must preserve all the energy that it has, so the metabolism slows down accordingly.

We know that in some of the Third World countries people can function and work well and hard on a diet of one bowl of rice per day. This is because the body has become attuned to this. The body's metabolism has slowed itself down to such an extent that a person can work quite healthily on such a low level of sustenance.

The same thing happens when a very low-calorie diet is followed. The body adjusts itself so that it can function on almost nothing. Unfortunately, when the dieter has reached the target weight and decides it is time to take some real nourishment, the weight lost is quickly regained and proves to be very difficult to lose again, even on a sensible diet, because the body has been taught to function on 400-500 calories per day. Anything exceeding this amount, even a modest 1,000 calories, will cause a weight gain.

If you have taught your body to accept 500 calories per day as being normal, then reverting to a 1,000-calorie slimming diet will mean that your body is receiving 500 calories per day more than it needs. This amounts to 35,000 calories per week, which corresponds to a pound of fat. Not only does the weight continue to pile on until you have reached your former weight, but, because the metabolism has been destroyed by this very low-calorie diet, you will keep gaining weight until you are far heavier than you were originally.

This is the least horrific effect that can occur after having been on a very low-calorie diet. Some poor unfortunates have had to be hospitalised because all their vital functions have slowed down to a virtual standstill. I treated a girl in our clinic not so long ago who had to be revived and brought back from death's door. Her bowels did not function, her liver did not function, her kidneys did not function — and it took a great deal of careful nursing to get this girl back on her feet again.

I saw this girl twice; neither time did she lose weight. I often wondered what happened to her after that. It really is most distressing for many people when they find that the old faithful 1,000-calorie diet on which they used to lose weight relatively easily no longer works for them. So, be very careful when a synthetic diet offers you the promise of substantial weight losses in a very short time. These promises will be realised; but consider the consequences.

In recent years many such diets have sprung up. There is the "Scarsdale" diet, which is a very one-sided protein diet. Indeed, you do lose a lot of weight, but it is not very healthy. There is the "Beverly Hills" diet, which allows you to eat great amounts of one sort of food at a time. Again you lose weight, but it is difficult to adhere to and proves very awkward when dining out. There are also the mad diets, like the "banana and milk" diet and the "cheese and champagne" diet. All these diets are one-sided and although a weight loss will be achieved, they are diets to be followed for a short time only; they cannot possibly be adhered to forever. Moreover, they are very unnatural and for that reason alone should be avoided.

What we ideally want to do is find a way of life that is pleasing to ourselves, but at the same time will not do our diet any harm. That is why we should not embark upon a crash diet. The sensible dieter may not experience enormous weight losses after the first few weeks, but *will* experience a gradual feeling of being satisfied with the good wholesome food that nature offers.

Many people think that they will lose a great amount of weight in a very short time if they go on a fast. Now, fasting in itself is not a bad thing, because it gives the body a rest and clears the system. It is a very good basis for starting a good, sensible new way of life. Again, though, the same happens as with a very low-calorie diet. The metabolism slows down to accommodate the starvation situation.

A water fast can be very difficult, so most people elect for a juice fast. Drink as much water as you can or want, but, in addition, two or three times a day, drink a glass of unsweetened fruit juice. Keep this up for two or three days and then, very gradually, start on a sensible eating plan.

Not everybody finds it easy or even possible to go on a fast. The first half day is the worst, after which it becomes easier. If you do not manage a fast before starting your new way of life, don't worry. Your revised lifestyle will soon give you a fresh feeling of well-being that you will speedily come to regard as normal.

Through reading this chapter, you will now realise that there are no short cuts to losing weight. Your aim must be not just to lose weight quickly, but to lose weight permanently. Have you ever considered the fact that if you lose one pound per week, that adds up to almost four stones per year?

Don't start your diet thinking, "I'll never again eat anything sweet or anything fatty. I'll never look at crisps or chocolates again." You will. Realise that you cannot win every battle, but you can achieve the ultimate victory.

Finally, remember the story of the hare and the tortoise. The hare, in spite of his great speed, did not win the race. It was the tortoise, with his slow, plodding, steadfastness that gained the prize.

11

Excuses

AS A GROUP dieters are the most imaginative people that I know. The range of excuses I have had to accept over the years for people not arriving for their appointments is quite phenomenal.

The most common, of course, is the "broken down car". They were half-way there when, alas, the car ceased to function! One lady who seems to have suffered a very great misfortune each time she has bought a car has attended our clinic for years. Each year, on 1 August, she buys a new car, but every other week the car seems to malfunction. She will ring up with the most obscure technical details about what exactly is wrong with it and why she couldn't keep her appointment, then the next time she comes I find that she has put on half a stone in weight, which of course was the real excuse. Also, the petrol in many cars seems to run out just short of reaching our clinic. What puzzles me is how the people in it managed to make it back home to phone me!

Dieters also tend to be singularly unfortunate with their health and the health of their families. This is another great excuse for not arriving. They were sick. They had a virus that was going around. They had such a cold that they couldn't possibly come. They were suffering from a migraine. If they weren't doing it, their husband was having a heart attack or had suddenly become paralysed!

It amazes me that there are any adults in this world when I think of the dreadful things that befall their children. They swallow a fortune in coins — and golf balls seem to be their staple diet! The falls that they suffer are beyond description, yet when one sees them the next time, accompanying their parents, they will appear to be perfectly healthy, in fact, quite ordinary little human beings.

One excuse for not losing weight that I hear regularly is the menstrual cycle. The dieter is either about to have a period, has just had a period or is in the middle of having one. Some people seem to be continually using these excuses each week. I often wonder what sort of body they have. Granted, there is little extra fluid in a normal person just before the menstrual cycle and sometimes even during ovulation, which occurs half-way between two periods, but mostly this is very temporary, so I don't really accept this as a valid excuse.

A great excuse, too, is provided by the workman who didn't turn up. It would appear that there are no reliable tradesmen left in Scotland. Inevitably, they will ring up and make an appointment with the client. The client then programmes her day around the arrival of the workman. She gives him perhaps five minutes leeway and then he doesn't turn up. He arrives ten minutes later and this provides a wonderful excuse for cancelling the slimming appointment.

Dieters also have a ball when the teachers go on strike. They forget that throughout the school holidays and in the evenings the waiting-room is crowded with children because the dieters have no babysitter. But when the schools are on strike the appointment cannot be kept because the dieters have to stay at home and attend to their offspring.

The telephone, too, provides a wonderful excuse when all else fails. Just as the dieter was about to leave the house, the telephone rang and it was a friend who had talked for hours. After she hung up, she realised it was far too late for her to keep her appointment. The lady completely ignores the fact that when it suits her she can arrive an hour late without so much as an explanation.

A traffic jam is another great excuse. I can travel anywhere and almost never become stuck in a traffic jam, but the traffic jams that appear to occur when I am sitting in my consulting-room seem to congest the whole of Scotland. Traffic lights frustrate many in their attempts to reach our clinic, but the fact that the set of traffic lights has always been there doesn't seem to come into it. It was there when the dieter was attempting valiantly to arrive at Auchenkyle, therefore she was far too late to keep her appointment!

These are the excuses I hear for people not turning up. I might add that some of these appointments are not even cancelled. The next time the dieter arrives, inevitably without an appointment, these are the excuses given to me.

Now come the excuses for not having lost weight or for having gained weight. The favourite one here is nibbling because of worry. The gained weight adds to the initial worry and, of course, the "vicious circle" is set in motion.

We have already gone into all this when looking at the reasons for gaining weight — worry, boredom and fear. However, the fact is that they are, when one really thinks about them, just excuses. Some of them are quite classic. Take Mrs X, for example:

Mrs X is a very nervous body, and her older children have reached the stage where they are at university and occasionally come home for a weekend, bringing a friend with them. Mrs X's son rang up and said he was arriving on Friday with a friend and that they were intending to spend the weekend. This, of course, sent Mrs X into a panic, and the ammunition for dealing with a panic was, of course, the biscuit tin! She munched her way through the biscuits and then rang up her son to say that she was in no fit state to receive visitors, therefore it would be better if he did not bring his friend with him. Her son was disappointed but agreed that perhaps his mother's health was not up to it. He said he would explain this to his friend who would fully understand the situation. Mrs X replaced the receiver and shakily made her way to the cake tin, since the biscuit tin was empty, and proceeded to demolish the contents of that. This crisis causes Mrs X to have a weight gain of three pounds.

When we analyse this scenario, we see that the whole panic was caused by the visit of a stranger who didn't even come. Perhaps if Mrs X had received her son's friend, she would have enjoyed the visit and have been so distracted that she would have stuck to her diet, being so busy cooking for the large appetites of young men that she would have little time to eat herself.

On the other hand, entertaining visitors can be, of course, a great excuse for not having lost, or even having gained, weight. One cannot expect one's visitors to enjoy food if the hostess is not prepared to eat along with them.

Moving house is another classic. People seem to move into a new house having no kitchen, no cooker, no gas or electricity and, having got there, they then proceed to live from the local fish and chip shop. This tends to continue for months on end and each time they come back to me they wonder why, in spite of the violent exercise they are doing in cleaning their house, each fortnight sees a weight gain.

Holidays, birthdays (including the cat's), Christmas and Easter, Ramadan, Jewish New Year and Chinese New Year are all great excuses for people of every persuasion to gain weight. Christians, Jews, Muslims and Hindus all very sympathetically share in each other's festive seasons. Since hardly a week goes by when there is nothing in the world to celebrate, some people are very hard pressed to lose even one pound.

Although some of these excuses are slightly exaggerated by me, I have heard them all, and I regularly meet people who use them. The one excuse that never fails to amuse me is the one made by the lady who suddenly stops her treatment and arrives perhaps a year or a year and a half later, the excuse being that she has been ill. I express, of course, great concern that anybody could be ill for such a long time, and ask her what the ailment was. Usually she had had a heavy head cold and therefore was unable to attend for year to a year and a half. When she does return, it is with, of course, the usual weight gain.

Some excuses are genuine and duly deserve sympathy. Most, however, are very transparent and not even particularly original. I hear the same excuses day in and day out, and I sometimes wonder why people bother to make excuses at all. Of course, some people don't make excuses; they just don't turn up, having failed to cancel their appointment. They then start attending again, two or three months later, expressing great surprise and disappointment, and frequently suggesting that it is somehow my fault that they have gained weight.

We have looked at the excuses and the people who make them. Now we come to the disbelievers. When these people enter the consulting-room and I ask them how they have got on, they will tell me that they have had a terrible fortnight and proceed to expound on all the dreadful things that they have done in terms of eating. Carefully stepping on the scales and hearing that they have gained a pound, they express extreme surprise at this and at the fact that the programme is not working. When I remind them of the confessions they have just made, they look surprised and say, "Oh, but I didn't cheat all that much and I have cut down, so why should I have gained a pound?" When I then point out that they are not really on a diet at all, unless they are doing exactly what I have told them, they start to argue with me.

Sometimes when I ask people how they have fared, they will look me straight in the eye and reply threateningly, "I have lost five pounds." That, of course, remains to be seen. I always take my scales to be the judge of how much a person has lost. The scales that I use do not work on a spring balance. They work on knife edges, therefore they are not influenced by variations in humidity or temperature, nor can the person using them lose a few pounds by standing on tip-toe on one foot. Their weight, when they stand on the scales, is accurately measured by the balancing of a knife. When I dare to disagree and tell them that they have not lost five pounds, but two pounds, I am met with all sorts of protestations. Theirs are new scales. They are computer scales. Their scales cannot possibly be wrong. My scales are wrong.

One of my daughters has a new set of scales. We tried them, standing in various positions and putting the scales in various positions on the floor. We managed to record a fluctuation of nine pounds. A friend of mine then acquired a set of computer scales. Again we tried them out in the same manner; this time we managed to record a fluctuation of six pounds.

Unless scales work on a knife edge and are properly balanced they will merely indicate a trend upwards or downwards of a person's weight. They are by no means accurate. It need not be important whether they are accurate or not. What really matters is whether you are becoming slimmer. Are your clothes becoming looser? Do you look better? Do you feel better? These are the true criteria.

I am not for a moment suggesting that dieting is easy, but what I do say is that if you have your priorities right, if you are really determined to lose weight, you will see every difficulty for what it is — just an excuse!

Some excuses are better than others. Some excuses are easier to understand than others. Some excuses must be dealt with very sympathetically. But whatever it is, if you fail to lose weight because you have not stuck to your diet, it is because you have found an excuse. The people who usually succeed the best in losing weight are the ones who admit that they have not lost weight on that particular occasion because they have been doing something that they should not have been doing. They do not attempt to make excuses for this. They realise it is hampering their weight loss but they understand and realise that unless they do exactly what they are told and sweep aside all excuses, they are not going to lose weight.

These people are the ones who are easier to help because they understand the situation completely and are willing to abide by the rules. If you make your own rules, the chances are that you will not lose weight, however valid the excuse for not sticking to your diet might be.

12

Useful Advice

AS I HAVE already observed, dieting is never easy. Some people, however, seem to set themselves up for failure before they have even begun. They go shopping and buy as if food was going out of fashion. Everything that they could possibly need is bought in one go. Much of it is very useful for people who are dieting; but on the other hand, if one has too much choice, then deciding what to eat at a given moment becomes very difficult and, especially if one is hungry, this often leads to too much being eaten at once. The diet then fails before it has even started.

In order to prevent this kind of thing happening to your diet, I will provide in this chapter a number of little tips which will help you through your daily life. A separate list is given for a number of situations which commonly give rise to problems, and these are followed by a list of general tips. As we have started by looking at "shopping", then the first of these lists deals with this subject.

Shopping
1. Never shop on an empty stomach. If one is hungry,

all sorts of temptations loom up in front of one at a supermarket.

2. Before you set off on a shopping expedition, make a list of the things you need and don't look at anything else.

3. Try to shop just once a week for the things on your list. If necessary, store them in the freezer.

4. Separate your own food from the food that you are going to buy for the family.

5. Do not buy your own favourite foods for the family. There are plenty of different foods on the market, so don't choose the ones that are going to tempt you the most when you go shopping for your family.

6. When you reach the check-out, try to concentrate on the person you are going to be once you are slim, and then you will not see all these tempting items most supermarkets keep just at the check-out.

Having done your shopping and returned home, the next danger area you will enter is the kitchen, so my second list is headed *In the Kitchen*.

In the Kitchen

1. Spend as little time as possible cooking. Don't go into the kitchen just to see what is there. Go in, do what you have to, then get out.

2. While you are cooking, do not taste the food. A teaspoonful leads to a dessertspoonful, which leads to a tablespoonful, which really leads to a whole "mini-meal" before you are even anywhere near the table. You know that your cooking is fine. You have been doing it for a long time, so there is no need to taste it!

3. For your particular diet, weigh all your food and then you know exactly what you are eating and how much.

4. Do not persuade yourself to be "roped into" baking or making toffee or fudge for good causes. There are enough things that you could be doing for good causes with your sewing machine or even helping to sell these things, but do not make them, because you know where some of it will go! There are enough people willing to do the cooking and baking who do not have a weight problem, or who are not interested in their weight. You do something else, or even make a contribution so that someone else can do the cooking or baking, but do not do it yourself!

5. Use cooking methods that do not entail a high number of calories. For example, food that is grilled is often much more tasty than food that is fried in a lot of fat. Avoid frying or deep frying as far as possible. Cook all your meat either by roasting, grilling or boiling. Be very aware of how much fat you use in your cooking. Also be very aware of how much sugar you use. These are the calories that mount up rapidly without being particularly good for you. Food tastes much better in its natural state, so don't try to disguise it with a lot of fat or too much sugar.

Many of my dieters go out to work. This again is fraught with danger for someone trying to lose weight. So, the next list concerns those who are out working away from home.

Out Working

1. Take a packed lunch with you. If you know exactly what is in your lunch then you know that you are sticking to your diet. Hotels, restaurants and canteens cannot be held responsible for your gaining weight at lunchtime.

2. It is a good idea to make your packed lunch well in advance. For example, perhaps on a Sunday evening you could make a week's supply of lunches in one fell swoop and then put them into the freezer. When you go out in the morning, take one packed lunch with you. It will not be thawed until lunchtime, so the temptation to eat it with your morning coffee will not arise.

3. When coffee-time arrives, do not be tempted by biscuits, scones, rolls or any other things that tend to fly around offices at that time of the day. Tell your colleagues what you are doing, and then you will not dare to take something that you shouldn't, in case they laugh at you.

4. When you have eaten your lunch at lunchtime, find something to do that interests you; otherwise you may be tempted to go to the canteen for just that little extra bit of something nice. Go window-shopping for clothes. Go into the library and read a book. Go for a walk. Do anything but expose yourself to extra food.

5. Do not keep sweets in a drawer. If you do that, then they will always be at the back of your mind and your will-power will fly out of the window. So, see that there are no sweets, crisps or anything else that might tempt you during working hours.

6. Beware of office parties. In some large offices every week there is at least one birthday party at lunchtime or at break-time. If you have told your colleagues what you are doing, I'm quite sure they will not hold it against you if you refuse their piece of cake, or their sticky bun, or whatever treat they have brought because it is their birthday.

Remember to refuse their offer politely, but not regretfully. If you say "no thank you" in a tone that really says "yes please" then you will be coaxed and inevitably you will be tempted and eventually accept the offering. If you are quite firm but still friendly, then they will realise that your intentions are serious. They in turn will take you seriously and help you.

For some people meal times at home present the greatest danger. Whether you are alone or in company, meal times can for some people be the cause of disaster. So, the next list is headed *Mealtimes*.

Mealtimes

1. Always, even when you are alone, eat at the table, sitting

in the same place. Eventually, you will come to regard this place as the only place in the house where you should eat. We have already talked about the habit-forming nature of human beings. This is one way in which you can use this to help yourself.

2. If you are having a hot meal, make your plate and your meal as hot as possible. This will help to slow down the rate at which you eat your food.

3. Chew your food well. The more you chew it, the longer it will last, and the more you will be satisfied, because if you eat slowly your stomach will tell you when you have had enough. If you eat too quickly, then although you have had enough, you will still feel hungry because your stomach has had no time to convey this full feeling as a message to the brain.

4. Put down your knife and fork between each mouthful. This is another way to make your meal last longer. If you eat it too quickly, then you will not feel you have had anything. This is where a hot plate and piping hot meal comes in handy. You do not need to rush to finish it before it is cold.

5. Do not read at the table. While you are reading, your mind is only partially concentrating on what you are eating; because of this, you eat mindlessly. You will then eat too quickly with the result yet again that you eat too much.

6. Eat your food from a smaller plate. Your meal will look more substantial if the plate is full. If your plate is too large, then your eye thinks that you are not having enough to eat. So, the fuller your plate, the more you are going to be satisfied with what you are eating.

7. Do not finish off the family left-overs. This is a habit that many people are guilty of. We all know about the starving millions, but your eating up what the family leaves does

not help them. All it does is add inches to your already too-thick thighs. If you have a dog or a cat, then there will be no waste and the problem is solved. If you have neither, then I'm afraid the only solution is to throw it away. It is waste, but perhaps in time you will learn that you are cooking too much food for your family. Cook them smaller meals if you constantly find that something is left over, but whatever happens do not put the left-overs in your mouth.

For some, having to socialise is the worst thing that can befall them. This need not be so. Remember, a social evening does not comprise solely of food. It is company. It is enjoying the company. It is enjoying the surroundings and the conversation. The food is provided just as a means of making these things more pleasant. If you can view socialising in this light, then you will get the food into the right perspective. One does not go out solely to eat, but one eats because one enjoys socialising with one's friends.

I have already talked about techniques when socialising, so I will not dwell on them. The following list is short and has already been expanded on earlier in the book.

Socialising

1. When you are in a hotel, choose your menu sensibly.

2. Remember to drink low-calorie and non-alcoholic drinks.

3. Keep your glass full so that it cannot be filled up again.

4. When you are eating make sure, especially at a friend's house, that you do not finish your meal first, then you are less likely to be offered a second helping.

5. If you are offered a second helping, do not accept it.

6. Do not nibble aimlessly. When one is socialising, there are often all sorts of little nibbles available, but nobody

minds if you do not partake of them.

For most people, the most difficult time of the day is the evening. They are in a relaxed mood, and feel that they should have some sort of reward for having got through the hazards, trials and tribulations of the day. For many dieters this reward means a treat that goes into the mouth. This list is therefore entitled *Evenings*.

Evenings

1. Try to fill each evening with something that interests you. If you are bored when you come home from work and decide to do the ironing or the washing, or clean the windows, then your mind will automatically turn to food. Find something that you think is stimulating, then your mind will be occupied in a more constructive manner.

2. It is good to get out in the evenings if possible. See if you can find an interesting evening class, or go swimming, or join a gymnastic or yoga class. I know that this is not always possible because there are times when nobody can look after your children, but perhaps one or two evenings in the week can be filled in this way.

3. If you are going to be at home in the evening, make sure that you have a nibble dish of food that you are allowed — food that is part of your diet — so that when you feel the urge to eat something, you are not spoiling a good day's work.

4. Keep something back and have it for supper. If you have something to look forward to, then the evening does not seem nearly so long. If you have your last meal at, say, six o'clock, and know that no bite of food must pass your lips before breakfast the next day, then the evening can be very, very long, especially if food is in the back of your mind the whole time.

5. One good way to resist temptation is to have a hot, luxurious bath and take a book with you.

6. If you feel really tempted, it sometimes helps to clean your teeth. The feeling of needing something, especially something sweet, will usually pass. The same applies to having a lemon drink. This tends to take away the need for sweet things.

The tips given so far, if you heed them, should see you through the day. They all sound very good advice, and so they are, but sometimes they are not so easily followed. Temptation will, and does, creep in, so the next section under the heading *Miscellaneous* will deal with such situations.

Miscellaneous

1. When you have broken your diet, do not think that all is lost. If you have had a bad morning, then talk to yourself quite firmly, but don't nag. This will just make you miserable. Don't try to starve yourself to make up for all the sins that you have committed, but just put them behind you and start afresh as soon as possible.

Don't, like Mrs X, when you break your diet on Monday, postpone your next dieting attempt for another week. Start right away with the next meal, and you will find that by the end of the week you will still have managed a weight loss.

2. The most discouraging part of any diet is when you come to a "plateau". This has already been discussed in Chapter 6. You must persevere. Stop weighing yourself for a while and start measuring yourself. If you are truly sticking to your diet, then you will be encouraged. Remember, it is what you look like that counts; it is the inches that you are losing that the world sees. They don't know every ounce that goes on or comes off your weight.

3. Do not be envious of your thin friends who tend to eat far more than you do and never seem to gain an ounce.

What these people are doing is storing up a fat future for themselves. At a later date they will be most distressed to find that they can no longer eat the way they have been doing and stay slim.

These people, when their sins catch up with them, will be far more miserable than you, poor soul, who has had to diet throughout your whole life to keep anywhere near in trim.

4. You will find that the outside world is not nearly so supportive of your diet as you think it should be. Dieting is a very psychological process, not just for the dieter, but for those around her. For some reason, your slim friends may be afraid that you might catch up with them. Therefore, when they see a little weight coming off, they will tell you that, "You are all right. You don't need to go any further. You are slim enough."

Your fat friends will be discouraging too. They see that you are doing what they ought to be doing, and there is a fair measure of sour grapes when they tell you that "You are looking haggard. It doesn't suit you. Your disposition was much better when you were fat."

Don't listen to either set of friends. You will find that your most supportive friends will be the ones who are trying to diet themselves. They will help and encourage you. They will be pleased with your weight losses, and you in turn must be pleased with theirs. People who are not dieting tend to be very unsympathetic, either because they are thin and don't want you to be thin, or because they are fat and don't want you to be thin.

5. Sometimes you will find yourself in a situation you have not planned for. Knowing that these situations will inevitably arrive, you must be ready for them at any given time. Sometimes you will have planned your diet for the whole day and, suddenly, a very attractive invitation arrives for the evening. You know what to do when socialising. Keep this knowledge always in the back of your mind, so that if you suddenly find yourself in a social

position which you had not reckoned on, don't let it take you by surprise. You know the routine. Switch to it and stick to it.

6. Every dieter has a special time, or two or three times, in the day when dieting is particularly difficult. These times take a person unawares, unless they know when to expect them.

The best way of dealing with this is by charting your whole day for a week. Write down everything that you eat, and each time that you feel tempted. Note the emotion accompanying the temptation, or the situation in which you found yourself when the temptation struck. After a week, if you look at your chart, you will find that there is a pattern in it. There were certain times, certain emotions, certain situations, that triggered off a potential binge.

When you have determined which emotions and situations are likely to be dangerous, you can then sit down and make a plan of campaign. How are you going to cope with them? If the problem is boredom, make sure that there is something to do at that time. If it is tension, try to do some relaxing exercises at that time. If it is hunger — genuine hunger — make sure that you have something to eat at that time, something that is already prepared and is part of your diet.

7. When you are hungry, exercise. It is a fallacy that exercise makes you yet more hungry. If you are active, then you will find that the last thing on your mind is food. Activity has an exhilarating effect on the emotions. You feel alive, you feel fresh, you feel good, and you don't want to spoil those feelings by being "bogged down" with food.

People only think that exercise makes them hungry. If you examine your feelings after having exercised, you will discover that, if you are honest, you had previously been conditioned to regard exercise as something that increases the appetite; whereas, in actual fact, the more one exercises, the less one wants to eat. So, don't be afraid of moving. Don't be afraid of being energetic or exercising. It will give you a new life and it will make you feel a lot better and much less hungry.

8. Finally, I must talk here about vegetables. On most diets these can be eaten freely; they certainly can on my diet. Some people seem to think that salad, like grapefruit, has a magical slimming quality. This is, of course, not true. Nevertheless, any vegetable prepared in any way, except by frying, will help your diet.

I find that one good stand-by, and an excellent one for taking with you as a packed lunch, is slimmer's soup. There is no end to the varieties you can have. Basically, the recipe that I use is the same for each soup. You start with a stock cube and you can add anything in the way of vegetables that you like into it. Put in a tin of tomatoes, or tomato juice, or vegetable juice, in order to give it some colour. Add to that anything you like: mushrooms, leeks, mixed vegetables. Don't be afraid of using herbs and spices, as they will give a richness to your vegetable soup.

When the vegetables are ready, the soup is ready. At this stage, if you want to make a cream soup, liquidise the mixture and add a little of your daily milk allowance. This will give you a feeling of eating a very rich soup; while in actual fact you can have as much of it as you like because it is very low in calories.

In winter, I find a very good way of making a satisfying vegetable soup is to take the stock cube and add to your stock as many diced vegetables, fresh or frozen, as you want. When the soup is ready, liquidise half of it. This will make the stock much thicker and will fool you into thinking that you are eating something substantial.

Whichever way you like your soup, it is always savoury and it is a good stand-by. You can have as much of it as you like, as many times a day as you like, so there is no excuse for saying, "I broke my diet because I was hungry."

13

The New You

SO FAR, THIS book has concentrated mainly on explaining the reasons why you may be fat and why you may be finding it difficult to lose weight. Hopefully, from reading this, you will have learned what you are doing wrong in your attempt to achieve a good weight loss.

Having read and absorbed all of this, the time for action has now arrived. Sitting, agreeing with what I have said and wishing that you were slim will get you nowhere, as I have already said.

The easiest way to begin your diet is by organising yourself. If you are organised, everything will fall into place. If you are not organised, you will find great difficulty in sticking to any diet.

At our clinic we have three great weapons to help us fight the battle against fat. The first one is treatment. For this we use acu-aids. These are placed on the ear and will do several things for you: they will balance the body (the yin and the yang); they will speed up your metabolism; and, when you press the point, you will find that they will also give you will-power. Just press the point, think about something else or, if it is possible, do something else, and you will find that you are very easily distracted. You will forget about what it was you were going to eat that you should not have.

Once the acu-aids have been placed in the ear, the point, having been stimulated, will work for two weeks. It is for this reason that we like our dieters to attend the clinic on a fortnightly basis. In this way they will enjoy the benefit of continual assistance and a continual speeding up of the metabolism caused by the use of acu-aids.

Of course, this in itself will not help. You cannot sit back and say, "I have had acu-aids in my ear, therefore I am going to become slim." Unfortunately, you will have to work at it, and the only way to get slim is by what you do not put in your mouth. In other words, you must eat less than the body needs to keep it at the weight it is at the moment — and the only way to do that is to follow a diet!

Our diet, we find, is a very successful one. It is not calorie controlled, but chemically controlled, i.e. it contains all the vitamins, minerals and trace elements that you need to keep your body functioning and to keep yourself healthy. At the same time, it does have a low enough calorie count to allow your body to lose weight.

The reason that you do not have to count calories on this diet is because we have already done it for you. The only thing that you have to do is weigh your food. Everything that you eat, with the exception of vegetables, must be weighed — not just once, but each and every time. Your eye is an excellent judge in this respect. It sees what you need to keep your body at its present weight.

So, if you follow our diet but neglect to weigh your food, you will look good, you will feel good, you will even lose inches because the acu-aids tend to pull one in, but, alas, you will not lose weight. The only way to lose weight yourself is to be accurate with your weighing of food. Let the scales judge and the body will lose weight automatically.

The next thing we offer our dieters is a course of herbal pills. These pills will help to reduce the appetite, making you feel less hungry. If you feel less hungry, you will not have the inclination to eat more than you should. That is all that these pills do. They are not vitamins. They are not magic. They are simply herbal appetite suppressors. As mentioned in Chapter 8 they are not addictive; nor do they have any side-effects.

This method always works, provided you work with it. We can make it very easy for you because we can make your fat burn more quickly. We can make you feel less hungry. We can make you feel less tempted. It is up to you, however, to stick to your diet, and it is the degree to which you do this that determines whether you are going to lose weight. It is what you put into it that you get out of it.

At the top of the diet sheet you will find a suggested day's menu. It should be stressed that this is just what it says — a suggestion. Underneath, there is a list of daily and weekly allowances, and this constitutes your diet. If you stick to your daily allowance and eat it within twenty-four hours, and eat your weekly allowance within seven days, then you are sticking to your diet. So, just organise this to fit in with your own lifestyle. Don't try to change your lifestyle, but you must change your eating habits.

For example, if you are working at lunchtime, take a weighed packed lunch with you. If you like something to eat before you go to bed at night, keep something back. If you are working during the night, take your diet over a twenty-four-hour period. If you are a nibbler, then you are allowed to nibble, as long as what you nibble is on the diet sheet and weighed as part of your allowance.

Don't take any fewer than three meals per day. If you want, you can have more — five, six, seven, even eight — but don't take any fewer than three because otherwise, if you take your allowance in one fell swoop, you will overload your stomach and your metabolism will not work.

I touched upon this at the beginning of the book; how the body burns food as calories. One large meal will lie there like a great log on an empty fire, and no amount of matches will get that log burning. What your body needs is light meals several times per day. Each time you eat, you speed up your metabolism slightly; so six small meals per day will give you this little extra boost six times per day, instead of the normal three.

Before you start, read the diet below carefully and get yourself organised. Shop for the things that you will want for the next few days. See to it that everything that you need is in the house, because if it is not, then that is when you will grab for the biscuit tin. See to it when you are out working that there is something ready to have when you come in. That does not mean to say that your hot meal has to be ready when you come home; but see to it that you have a nibble dish in the fridge consisting of various sorts of vegetables, again so that you will not automatically turn to the biscuit tin.

Weight reduction diet

Suggested day's menu

Breakfast: Grapefruit or unsweetened fruit juice
Egg (poached, boiled, scrambled, omelette)
1 oz. wholewheat bread or toast, plus
butter from weekly allowance

Mid-morning: Tea or coffee

Lunch: Lean meat, fish, egg, cheese
Vegetables or salad
1 oz. wholewheat bread, plus butter from
weekly allowance (or exchange)
Fresh fruit (one portion)
Tea or coffee

Mid-afternoon: Tea or coffee

Evening meal: Clear vegetable soup or tomato juice
Lean meat, fish, egg, cheese
Vegetables or salad

1 oz. wholewheat bread, plus butter from weekly allowance (or exchange)
Fresh fruit (one portion)
Tea or coffee

Bedtime: Tea or coffee

Allowances
Daily: Milk (fresh) ½ pint or Marvel 1 pint
Wholewheat bread — 3 oz.
Meat— 4 oz. or Fish — 6 oz.
Fruit — three portions

Weekly: Butter or margarine — ¼ lb.
Cheese – ½ lb.
Eggs — seven (optional)

Exchanges for 1 oz. bread
Potato — one medium
Crispbread, crackers, water biscuits — two
Breakfast cereal — 1 oz., any sort except sugar-coated
Cooked rice — two dessertspoons
Plain biscuits or oatcakes — two

Variety is the spice of life — choose your allowances from these foods
Meats:
(4 oz. daily, cooked any way except fried)
Beef, chicken, corned beef, duck, kidney, lamb, liver, mutton, rabbit, sweetbread, tongue, tripe, turkey, veal

Fish:
(6 oz. daily, cooked any way except fried)
Cod, crab, haddock, halibut, hake, herring, kippers, lobster, ling, mackerel, mussels, oysters, pilchards, prawns, salmon, sardines, shrimps, trout, tuna

Eggs:
(Seven per week)
Poached, boiled, scrambled, omelette

Cheese:

BY APPOINTMENT ONLY

(1 oz. daily)
Caerphilly, Camembert, Cheddar, Cheshire, cottage (4 oz.), Danish Blue, Edam, Gruyère, Leicester, Parmesan, Roquefort, Stilton, Wensleydale, smoked Austrian

Vegetables:
(Unlimited)
Artichokes, asparagus, aubergines, bean sprouts, Brussels sprouts, beetroot, broccoli, cabbage (red, savoy, spring, winter), cauliflower, celery, carrots, cress, cucumber, courgettes, chicory, lettuce, marrow, mushrooms, onions, red and green peppers, pimentos, parsnips, parsley, French and runner beans, radishes, swedes, spring onions, spinach, pickles (dill, gherkins, red cabbage), tomatoes

(In moderation)
Peas, beans (butter, broad, haricot), sweetcorn, half avocado, baked beans (3.5 oz.)

Fruits:
(3 portions daily)

Apple, one average	Peach, one average
Apricots, two fresh	Pear, one average
Banana, one small	Pineapple, one slice fresh
Blackberries, 4 oz.	Plums, two
Cooking apples, one large (baked or stewed)	Pomegranate, one
	Raisins, 1 oz.
Cherries, 4 oz.	Raspberries, 4 oz.
Dates, 1 oz.	Rhubarb, 4 oz.
Damsons, ten	Strawberries, 4 oz.
Gooseberries, ten	Sultanas, 1 oz.
Grapefruit, one large	Tangerines, two
Grapes, 3 oz.	Unsweetened juice, 4 oz.
Melon, one slice	Orange, one average

Drinks:
Tea, Russian tea, herb tea, coffee, Bovril, Oxo, Marmite, soda water, PLJ, tomato juice, water, Energen 1 Cal.,

slimline drinks, low-calorie tonic

Seasonings:
Salt, pepper, vinegar, mustard, lemon juice, herbs, spices, Worcester sauce

These foods are best avoided
Sugar and its products:
Glucose, sweets, chocolate, ice-cream, sweetened yoghurt, jam, marmalade, lemon curd, treacle, syrup, puddings, lemonade, squashes, proprietary milk drinks, tinned fruits

Fatty foods:
Dripping, lard, oil, salad cream, cream, fat of meat, sausages, fried foods, black pudding, fishcakes, fish fingers, rissoles, chips, roast potatoes, potato crisps

White flour and its products:
Cakes, sweet biscuits, pastries, crumpets, doughnuts, scones, buns, dumplings, pies, bridies, sausage rolls, spaghetti, macaroni, thick gravies and sauces, thick pickles and chutneys, tinned packet soups, thick soups (peas, beans, lentils, barley, rice flour)

Miscellaneous items:
Honey, nuts, alcohol, evaporated or condensed milk, sorbitol, slimming biscuits, diabetic foods and squashes, processed meats

Many people come to me maintaining that they cannot lose weight, the excuse being "I work" or "I work at nights", or "the canteen at work doesn't cater for slimmers". These are feeble excuses. If you work, you are one of the privileged ones. If you work at night, then it doesn't matter. Your daily allowance allows you to take your diet over a twenty-four-hour period. You must have a meal at night, otherwise while you are working your blood sugar will become too low, and then you will not be able to work responsibly. Of course, the canteen at work cannot be held responsible for your failure to lose weight. You are responsible for this, so don't blame the canteen. Don't go to it. When you are out working, take a weighed meal with you, so that you know exactly what you are consuming.

Some people see obstacles everywhere, and they generally find that they do not lose weight. They are so busy looking at the difficulties that they forget to do their simple part of organising themselves so that the weight will fall off automatically.

There was one dieter who came to our clinic, and who I have not seen for a few years because he has kept his weight down, whom I admire tremendously. He was a lorry driver and did long-distance driving. He left the house every Sunday at half-past seven and did not arrive back home until the following Friday evening. He took everything that he needed for the whole week with him, including his dog and his football. Like other drivers, he stopped on the motorways for a rest, but he did not make use of the restaurant facilities. He had all his meals with him. He even kept a fridge in the lorry. He and his dog would also enjoy a game of football two or three times every day. This man amazed me. Each week he came with a good weight loss. He had found a new way of life, in spite of having a job that consisted of sitting for at least eight hours per day, five days per week. This man had a very active life in between his driving, and he completely changed his lifestyle and eating pattern. He has now kept this up for quite a few years, and I don't see any sign of him falling by the wayside.

There is one category of people who are at the mercy of others, but I have dealt with several of them and all have managed to do well. I am referring to those who work on the oil rigs. These people have every meal cooked for them, but these meals have been worked out by a dietician so that each worker receives what is estimated to be the average amount of food that one needs for the heavy work being done on these rigs. What makes many of these men gain a lot of weight is the fact that they are bored. They have long working hours, but there is nothing else to do but work. When they are not working they tend to go to the bar and spend their evenings drinking. Now this is a sure way of putting on a great amount of weight.

Most of these people who come to me have managed, by being careful with what they eat, by avoiding alcoholic drinks in the bar, and by keeping up some form of exercise, although this is not really necessary when doing hard manual labour, to decrease their weight by taking advantage of their periods at home. When they are at home they stick rigidly to the diet, and when they are on the rig they let their eyes judge and do not eat rubbish, so that their weight tends to come off in chunks rather than slowly, a pound or two per week. When they are at home they lose weight, and when they are away they maintain it; thus, each time they come home, another chunk comes off which is maintained until the next time.

I have already mentioned people who live largely in hotels because of their work. This, as I have said before, need not be a problem. True, you cannot weigh your food, but you can choose sensibly. When you are at home, stick rigidly to your diet and you, too, will find that you will manage a good weight loss.

Now let us see what Mrs X is doing.

She is very pleased with herself because she has managed to get a full-time job. The children were at school and her husband was out the whole day long, so she was bored. She felt that this was keeping her weight up, so a full-time job seemed to be the answer. She realised that she must have everything organised, otherwise she would never stick to her diet. For the first week or two this went pretty well.

On Saturday, Mrs X went shopping and bought enough food for the household for the whole week. Sunday evening saw her making sandwiches for the children's packed lunch at school, and for her own packed lunch at the office. She put them all in the freezer and was very pleased with herself at this idea because if she took one packed lunch out every day she knew she could not eat it before lunchtime because it would take that amount of time to thaw.

She prepared the meals in advance as far as was possible, so that everything was under control. However, the pressure of work, and home, and children, and cooking, very quickly got on top of Mrs X. Gradually, she started to buy a sandwich, and the sandwich became a roll, and the filling in the roll became progressively higher in calories. In the evening, she was so exhausted that the first thing she did, instead of having just a cup of coffee, was to have a cup of coffee with a biscuit before starting to prepare the evening meal. She picked her way through this cooking process and by the time the meal was on the table her excuse was that she was too tired to eat, but in reality she was too full to eat. She had already eaten several meals. No wonder poor Mrs X's weight went up!

There had to be a solution, so she found one. Her mother, who lives round the corner, volunteered to get the family meal ready in the evening. Mrs X started her diet again and told her mother that her portion of food must be weighed. She started, full of enthusiasm yet again, to take a packed lunch with her to work. In the evening her mother had the meal ready. It was a great luxury, but, alas, instead of following Mrs X's instructions, her mother neglected to weigh the food and, what is more, Mrs X became very tempted with all the extras that her mother had made for the children and her husband, so she helped herself to these as well. Her excuse when she came to me was, "Oh, my mother cooks for me and she doesn't weigh the food."

Now, make no mistake: nobody is responsible for your fat except yourself. You inflicted this upon yourself. It's your fat. You have put it on, and it's your responsibility and your responsibility alone to take it off. It's no good blaming those around you. It's no good blaming the circumstances under which you work. It's no good blaming the life you lead. These are all excuses. If your priority is to become slim, then these excuses will be very easily swept aside. If you do not really want to become slim, if you are half-hearted, then these excuses will loom as mountains high above you, and you will not be able to climb over them. Remember, going through the motions of sticking to a diet will never lead to success.

Several times per year I am confronted by ladies who say that they cannot eat everything that is on the diet sheet. This, considering their weight, is not very credible. When I ask these ladies what they have eaten, they say, "Oh, I stuck to the diet at the top of the sheet." However, if you look at the top of the sheet, there is nothing to say that this is a diet. It says that it is a *suggested day's menu*. What these ladies had been doing was methodically going through every item of food on every line, so that for lunch they had lean meat, fish, egg, cheese, vegetables or salad, one ounce of bread plus butter, fresh fruit, and tea and coffee. Now, this adds up to a large lunch. Of course everything was neatly weighed: four ounces of meat, six ounces of fish, one egg and one ounce of cheese. Imagine eating all that, and then going on to a dinner of four ounces of meat, six ounces of fish one egg, and cheese! When I pointed out to these ladies that their real diet was to be worked out from their daily and weekly allowances, they were less enthusiastic.

This is a good example of going through the motions of being on a diet, and will be very unsuccessful. Not only will it be unsuccessful but, because you think you are on a diet, then you feel that you are unable to lose weight and get depressed. Very carefully, do exactly what you are told, and your weight will come off. Don't eat anything that is not on the diet. Don't add anything to it and don't substitute. Do exactly what is on the diet and you will, it is guaranteed, lose weight.

BY APPOINTMENT ONLY

You have been left with no excuses. Start now. Use your imagination. Spend the time that you would otherwise spend eating in cooking imaginative meals for yourself. Dieting need not be a bore. It must become a way of life. So start now and have fun!

Useful Addresses

Bioforce (UK) Ltd
South Nelson Industrial Estate
Cramlington
Northumberland
NE23 9HL

Tel: (0670) 736537

Nature's Best Health Products Ltd
PO Box 1
1 Lamberts Road
Tunbridge Wells
TN2 3EQ

Tel: (0892) 34143

Auchenkyle
Southwoods Road
Troon
Ayrshire
Scotland
KA10 7EL

Tel: (0292) 311414

Index